TABLE OF CONTENTS

Top 20 Test Taking Tips

1. Carefully follow all the test registration procedures
2. Know the test directions, duration, topics, question types, how many questions
3. Setup a flexible study schedule at least 3-4 weeks before test day
4. Study during the time of day you are most alert, relaxed, and stress free
5. Maximize your learning style; visual learner use visual study aids, auditory learner use auditory study aids
6. Focus on your weakest knowledge base
7. Find a study partner to review with and help clarify questions
8. Practice, practice, practice
9. Get a good night's sleep; don't try to cram the night before the test
10. Eat a well balanced meal
11. Know the exact physical location of the testing site; drive the route to the site prior to test day
12. Bring a set of ear plugs; the testing center could be noisy
13. Wear comfortable, loose fitting, layered clothing to the testing center; prepare for it to be either cold or hot during the test
14. Bring at least 2 current forms of ID to the testing center
15. Arrive to the test early; be prepared to wait and be patient
16. Eliminate the obviously wrong answer choices, then guess the first remaining choice
17. Pace yourself; don't rush, but keep working and move on if you get stuck
18. Maintain a positive attitude even if the test is going poorly
19. Keep your first answer unless you are positive it is wrong
20. Check your work, don't make a careless mistake

NBCOT Information

1. You are allowed 4 hours for the NBCOT examination.There are 200 questions on the examination, however, only 170 questions are scored.
2. Each area of basic knowledge is not included with a specific block. All of the material is random. You will be required to "switch gears" between each of the above content areas.
3. If you take a break during the exams the testing clock will continue to count down.
4. The NBCOT is offered on the computer.
5. In many questions the occupational therapist or COTA must defer treatment and seek additional medical testing.
6. Remember the phrase Do No Harm and apply it to the testing situation involving patient care. Also a patient's airway should almost always be the first concern in an emergency.

Registering/Scoring for the NBCOT Licensure Test

Candidate Handbook
http://www.nbcot.org/WebArticles/articlefiles/40-2004%20Domestic%20Handbook.pdf

Scoring Breakdown
http://www.nbcot.org/WebArticles/articlefiles/139-scoring_and_reporting.pdf

National Board for Certification in Occupational Therapy
http://www.nbcot.org

National Board for Certification in Occupational Therapy, Inc.
The Eugene B. Casey Building
800 South Frederick Avenue
Suite 200
Gaithersburg, MD 20877-4150
(301) 990-7979
Fax (301) 869-8492

Neurology Review

The nervous system is made of the central nervous system (CNS) and the peripheral nervous system (PNS). The central nervous system is made up of the brain and the spinal cord. The peripheral nervous system consists of cranial and spinal nerves that innervate organs, muscles and sensory systems. The brain controls: thought, reasoning, memory, sight, and judgment. The brain is made up of four lobes: frontal, parietal, temporal, and occipital. The spinal cord is a made up of neural tracts that conduct information to and from the brain.

Cranial nerves in the peripheral nervous system connect the brain to the head, neck and truck. Peripheral nerves allow control of muscle groups in the upper and lower extremities and sensory stimulation. The peripheral nerves are spinal nerves that branch off the spinal cord going toward organs, and muscles.

The autonomic nervous system controls reflexive functions of the brain. Including "fight or flight" response and maintaining homeostasis. Homeostasis is a state of equilibrium within tissues. The autonomic nervous system uses neurotransmitters to help conduct nerve signals and turn on/off various cell groups.

Nervous tissue is composed of neurons, which are the functional unit of the nervous system. A neuron includes a cell body, and organelles usually found in cells. Dendrites provide receptive information to the neuron and a single axon carries the information away.

Key Terms:
Synapse- junction between two neurons
Action potential- threshold at which neurons fire

Brain

Frontal lobe-controls emotions, judgments, controls motor aspects of speech, primary motor cortex for voluntary muscle activation
Parietal lobe-receives fibers with sensory information about touch, proprioception, temperature, and pain from the other side of the body
Temporal lobe-responsible for auditory information, and language comprehension
Occipital lobe- center for visual information. Damage to the occipital lobes can result in disturbances of visual input, such as visual field cut or visual agnosia, in which objects can be seen but not recognized.
Cerebellum- coordination of muscle function. The cerebellum is located under the occipital lobes, and controls balance as well as smooth, coordinated movements. It is also active in motor memory. Damage to the cerebellum can result in ataxia, which is movement that is jerky and uncontrolled. Balance and equilibrium will also be affected, which will cause staggering. This is also known as ataxic gait.
Brainstem - (midbrain, pons, and medulla)-respiratory and cardiac center, nerve pathways to the brain. The brainstem includes the midbrain, the pons and the medulla. It is responsible for regulating the autonomic vital systems, such as controlling spontaneous breathing and the muscles of the heart. It also plays a role in eye movements and expression. Patients with damage in this part of the brain may experience vertigo or hearing loss, in addition to difficulties with swallowing.
Limbics system - The limbic system includes the cingulate gyrus of the cortex and the hippocampus. It is tucked into the midbrain, and connects to the frontal and temporal lobes. The limbic system is responsible for emotion, and some aspects of mapping and memory. The exact way in which limbic system regulates these two is not clear. Damage to the limbic system can result in long-term memory loss as well as emotional disturbances.
Diencephalon – *(thalamus, subthalamus, and hypothalamus)*
Thalamus – Integrate and relay sensory information from the face, retina, cochlea, and taste receptors. (Interprets sensation of touch, pain and temperature).

Hypothalamus

- Sleeping Cycle
- Controls the autonomic nervous system and the neuroendocrine systems.
- Maintains body homeostasis
- Thirst Center

- Helps regulate body temperature
- Helps regulate appetite control
- Thirst Center
- Control of Hormone secretion

Brain and spinal reflexes

- Spinal level reflexes are automatic motor responses to stimuli, and include flexor withdrawal, extensor thrust and crossed extension. Each of these reflexes is present from birth to two months, and assists with development of mobility patterns.
- Brainstem level reflexes automatic, are present from birth to 4 or 6 months, and are related to posture and initiation of the vestibular system. Examples of these include asymmetrical and symmetrical tonic neck reflex, tonic labyrinthine reflex, and positive supporting reaction.
- Midbrain reflexes develop from birth to 6 months, and are related to righting reactions and development of motor milestones. These include neck righting, labyrinthine righting on the head, body righting on the head and body righting on the body.
- Cortical reflexes are present through life, and involve communication between brain centers for touch, vision and the vestibular system. These include optic righting, and equilibrium reaction.

Glasgow Coma Scale

+Eye Opening
+Best Motor Response
+Best Verbal Response
Total (3-15 Score Range) A score of 1 in each category indicates no performance of skill.

Galveston Orientation and Amnesia test

A measure of orientation and memory, which is tallied to give a total score of up to 100. In this test, a patient is asked a series of ten questions and is given points for correct responses. An incorrect response results in a weighted deduction of points. Re-assessment can measure changes in cognitive status. This is a simple, quick measure of orientation.

Rancho Level of Cognitive Functioning Scale (LCFS)

The LCFS is one of the earlier developed scales used to assess cognitive functioning in post-coma patients. It was developed for use in the planning of treatment, tracking of recovery, and classifying of outcome levels. Use of the scale generates a classification of the patient in one of eight levels:
- Level I: "No Response" in which the patient does not respond to any stimuli.
- Level II: "Generalized Response" in which there is only non-specific and non-purposeful response to stimuli.
- Level III: "Localized Response" in which there is inconsistent and/or delayed response, specifically related to stimuli.
- Level IV: "Confused-Agitated" in which there is heightened response to stimuli, and severe confusion with possible agitation.
- Level V: "Confused-Inappropriate" in which there is response to simple commands and confusion with complex commands. The patient is easily distracted.

- Level VI: "Confused-Appropriate" in which responses are goal-directed, though cues may be necessary.
- Level VII: "Automatic-Appropriate" in which responses are goal-directed and appropriate but memorized, with decreased judgment and problem solving.
- Level VIII: "Purposeful-Appropriate" in which responses are adequate, though mild impairments are still present.

Autonomic Nervous System

Sympathetic (Fight or Flight):
1. Dilated pupils
2. Elevates heart rate and respiratory rate
3. Sweating
4. Epinephrine and norepinephrine secreted
5. Increased blood pressure
6. Constriction of skin and abdominal arterioles

Parasympathetic:
1. Constricted pupils
2. Lowers heart rate and respiratory rate
3. Increased peristalsis
4. Acetylcholine secreted
5. Decreases blood pressure
6. Relaxation of skin and abdominal arterioles

Cranial Nerves

I.   Olfactory nerve: sends an impulse to the brain relating to the sense of smell.
II.   Optic nerve: sends an impulse to the brain relating to visual discrimination and visual field.
III.   Oculomotor nerve: motor fibers send impulses to the muscles that control lens shape as well as inward and vertical eye movement. Sensory fibers send impulses to the brain that assist with proprioception of the eyes.
IV.   Trochlear nerve: motor fibers send impulses to the muscles that control downward and inward movements of the eyes.
V.   Trigeminal nerve: motor and sensory fibers send impulses for sensation in the mouth, nose and eyes as well as motor impulses for jaw movement and the muscles that control eating.
VI.   Abducens nerve: motor fibers send impulses to the muscles that control outward eye movements.
VII.   Facial nerve: motor and sensory fibers send impulses to and from the tongue, as well as the muscles that control expression.
VIII.   Vestibulocochlear: sensory fibers send impulses to the brain for hearing and equilibrium.
IX.   Glossopharyngeal nerve: motor fibers send impulses to the salivary glands, and sensory fibers send signals to the brain for bitter, sweet and sour.
X.   Vagus nerve: motor and sensory fibers send impulses to and from the larynx and the pharynx. Fibers also travel to and from the viscera of the abdominal organs and the parasympathetic system.
XI.   Spinal accessory nerve: motor and sensory fibers travel to and from the muscles that allow movement in the neck and shoulders.

XII.   Hypoglossal nerve: motor and sensory fibers travel to and from the tongue for its movement and proprioception.

Decorticate vs. Decerebrate Rigidity

Decorticate posturing-Upper limbs in flexion and the lower limbs in extension
Decerebrate posturing- Increased tone with all limbs in a position of extension

Circle of Willis Arteries

1   Lateral striate
2   MCA- middle cerebral artery
3   PCA- posterior communicating artery
4   Anterior communicating artery
5   Anterior cerebral artery

CVA, Stroke

1. Anterior cerebral stroke: lower extremity more involved than upper extremity, contralateral hemiparesis and sensory deficits
2. Posterior cerebral stroke: contralateral sensory loss, transient contralateral hemiparesis
3. Middle cerebral artery stroke: upper extremity more involved than the lower extremity, contralateral sensory loss
4. The right hemisphere of the brain controls movement and interprets sensation on the left side of the body. A CVA on this side of the brain will affect motor skills and sensation in the left upper and lower extremities. The patient may be emotionally labile, and may have difficulty processing visual-spatial information. Interpretation of abstract information and the non-verbal components of communication may be impaired. Attention span may be decreased, and left neglect or inattention may be present.
5. The left hemisphere of the brain controls movement and interprets sensation on the right side of the body. A CVA here will interrupt these pathways. Speech may be affected, including reception and processing of verbal and auditory information. Receptive or expressive aphasia may be present. The patient may also have a decreased right visual field.

Impairments Related to CVA
1. Constructional apraxia is the inability to perform actions on objects that require assembly. A patient with this condition might not be able to put toothpaste on his toothbrush, but could carry out the action of brushing his teeth.
2. Ideomotor apraxia is the inability to follow a motor command to completion. The individual might understand the directions given; however, he will not be able to physically finish the task.
3. Homonymous hemianopsia is a right or left field cut in both eyes, obscuring one complete side of the visual field. This is often coupled with unilateral neglect.
4. Nonfluent aphasia is difficulty with speech production, and is often linked with agraphia, which is the inability to express thoughts on paper. This speech is often stuttered and filled with pauses as the patient seeks the intended words.

Risk Factors
1. Diabetes

2. Atherosclerosis
3. Hypertension
6. Cardiac disease
7. Transient ischemic attacks

Aneurysm Precautions
1. Avoid rectal temperatures
2. Limit visitors
3. Avoid Valsalva's maneuver
4. Head of bed should be between 30-45 degrees

Valsalva's maneuver –causes an increase in intrathoracic pressure with an accompanying collapse of the vein of the chest wall. The following may result:
1. Decreased return of blood to the heart
2. Slowing of the pulse
3. Elevated intrathoracic pressure

Disorders

Autonomic Dysreflexia- caused by a lesion in the high thoracic or cervical cord. Severe hypertension, sweating and headaches noted. May occur with a blockage in a urine catheter.
Signs/Symptoms
1. Bradycardia
2. Headache
3. Increased parasympathetic activity
4. Excessive perspiration
5. Excessive sympathetic response
6. Elevated blood pressure
7. Stimulation of baroreceptors in aortic arch and caroticd sinus

Parkinson's Disease-a degenerative disease with primary involvement of the basal ganglia; characterized by the following:
Signs/Symptoms
1. Bradykinesia
2. Resting tremor
3. Impaired postural reflexes
4. Rigidity
5. Loss of inhibitory dopamine
6. Mask like affect
7. Emotional lability

Post-polio Syndrome- slowly progressive muscle weakness disease seen in individuals who survive the poliomyelitis virus, often in childhood.
Signs/Symptoms
1. Onset of muscle Weakness
2. Pain/Myalgia
3. High levels of fatigue

Multiple Sclerosis–progressive demyelinating disease of the central nervous system affecting mostly young adults and is chronic.
Cause unknown, most likely viral.

1. Fluctuating exacerbations
2. Demyelinating lesions limit neural transmission
3. Confirmed with lumbar puncture, elevated gamma globulin, CT/MRI, myelogram, EEG.
4. Mild to moderate impaired cognition common
5. Sensory Deficits
6. Bowel and Bladder Deficits
7. Spasticity common
8. Ataxic gait

Myasthenia gravis- neuromuscular disease characterized by fatigue of skeletal muscles and muscular weakness.
Signs/Symptoms

1. Progressive involvement
2. Decreased muscle membrane acetylcholine receptors
3. Severe weakness (proximal more than distal muscles)
4. Facial, ocular and bulbar weakness
5. Possible life-threatening respiratory muscle weakness
6. Probable use of anticholinesterase drugs for treatment

Guillain-Barre' Syndrome-polyneuropathy with progressive muscular weakness
Signs/Symptoms

1. Demyelination of peripheral and cranial nerves
2. Motor paralysis in an ascending pattern
3. 3% Mortality – respiratory failure
4. Autonomic dysfunction-arrhythmias, blood pressure changes, tachycardia

Amyotrophic lateral sclerosis (Lou Gehrig's disease) – degenerative disease that affects anterior horn cells and corticospinal tracts.
Signs/Symptoms

1. Death typically in 2-5 yrs.
2. Spasticity, hyperreflexia
3. Dysarthria, Dysphagia
4. Autonomic Dysfunction in approximately 1/3 of patients
5. Cognition is normal

Appropriate OT Interventions::
Initially the patient with ALS will present as independent in all aspects of self-care, however might exhibit mild weakness. In this stage, ROM and exercise are encouraged. As muscles begin to weaken, it is appropriate to introduce energy conservation and work simplification techniques including the use of adaptive equipment as appropriate. As the patient becomes non-ambulatory, assistive devices should focus on use from the wheelchair level. ROM remains appropriate at this stage, though should be passive in the muscles which are most affected. Patients should also be educated on pressure relief to prevent skin breakdown as the ability to weight shift becomes impaired. In the final stages, the patient and family members should be advised on use of home equipment and necessary environmental modifications, in addition to body mechanics training to prevent caregiver injury. Passive ROM is still appropriate, as is pain management and positioning for comfort.

Muscular dystrophy- group of very similar genetic diseases, characterized by a progressive weakening of the muscles.

Signs/Symptoms

Weakening of skeletal muscle.

Organs can also be affected, including the digestive system, the skin and the heart. Decreased range of motion.

Scoliosis is common.

Prognosis depends on the severity of the disease, which is sometimes fatal as early as childhood.

Seizures

Epilepsy-recurrent seizures due to excessive and sudden discharge of cerebral cortical neurons.

Tonic-clonic (Grand Mal) –Pt. confused and drowsy about the seizures, 2-5 min generally

Absence seizures (Petit Mal)- Brief, no convulsive contractions, may be up to 100X day

Simple Seizures- no loss of consciousness

Complex Seizures, brief loss of consciousness with psychomotor changes

**Key Point- When a patient has a seizure during most interventions, do not use a tongue blade and allow free movement in a safe environment

Meningitis-inflammation of the meninges of the spinal cord and brain caused by bacteria.

The most common bacteria are the following: *Neisseria meningitidis, Diplococcus pneumoniae,* and *Haemophilus influenzae*

Signs/Symptoms
1. Brudzinski's sign
2. Kernig's sign
3. Stiff/Tight neck
4. Fever
5. Confused

Horner's Syndrome- A lesion in the brain stem that causes disrupted sympathetic innervation to the face and causes: no sweating, ptosis and papillary constriction.

Upper Motor Neuron Lesion- occur within the motor tracts of the brain and/or spinal cord (CNS). Patients with these types of lesions will have a loss of voluntary muscle control and may experience increased tone, or spasticity, in the affected muscles. There will be an increase in deep tendon reflexes, and clonus may be present.
- Disuse atrophy
- +Babinski
- Hypertonia (Spasticity)
- Weakness or paralysis of movement not individual muscles
- Hyperreflexia

Lower Motor Neuron Lesion- occur in the axons or cell bodies of the peripheral nerves including those located in the brainstem and anterior horn of the spinal cord. Patients with these types of lesions also have a loss of muscle control, but demonstrate decreased muscle tone, or flaccidity. Deep tendon reflexes will be decreased or absent, and the associated muscles will atrophy. The patient may possibly be at risk for contracture if there is overpowering of the unaffected muscles in the affected limb.
   A. True Atrophy

B. Weakness of individual muscles
C. Fibrillations
D. Hyporeflexia

APGAR score: (Appearance, Pulse, Grimace, Activity, Respiration) (0-2) each category.
1. Color
2. Heart Rate
3. Reflex irritiability
4. Muscle tone
5. Respiratory effort

Reflex Arc

The typical pathway of a reflex may be outlined as follows: sensory receptor on dendrite of dorsal root ganglion cell --------→ ganglion cell ----------→ axon cell --------→ dorsal root --------→dorsal horn of spinal cord--------→ either directly to motor cell in ventral horn or via internuncial (association) neuron to ventral horn motor cell-------→ axon via ventral root ------→ spinal nerve-------→ effector organ (e.g., muscle).

Brunnstrom Stroke Recovery Stages:
1. No voluntary movement, Initial flaccidity and no tone noted.
2. Onset of hyperreflexia, synergies and spasticity
3. Movement in synergy
4. Decrease in synergy, some voluntary motor control
5. Progressing improvement with voluntary motor control
6. Patient has returned to semi-normal state- near normal

PNF Terminology:
Contract-relax
Agaonist reversals
Alternating isometrics
Hold-Relax
Rhythmic initiation
Resisted progression

Types of Memory

Immediate memory is the ability to recall information provided within the last minute. A patient with a deficit in immediate memory might be unable to follow directions completely, or may forget what the therapist has just taught them.
Delayed memory is the ability to recall information from up to a few hours previous. A patient with a deficit in this area might forget what happened during treatment an hour ago.

Procedural memory refers to the ability to recall the motor components for completing a task. An example of a deficit in procedural memory would be a patient who has forgotten how to ride a bike.

Prospective memory is the ability to self-cue for future performance of activities. An example of a deficit in prospective memory would be forgetting to take evening pills from a pillbox that has already been laid out.

Spinal Tracts

Ascending Pathways in the Posterior Funiculus

Fasciculus Gracicilis and Fasciculus Cuneatus - These pathways convey information on two point discrimination, vibration, and concious proprioception from nerves in the dorsal root ganglion to the ipsilateral nucleus gracilis and nucleus cuneatus, respectively, in the medulla oblongata where they synapse with secondary neurons. Fibers entering the tracts are added laterally and fibers originating in the lumbrosacral region are located most medially. The fasciculus gracilis is located medially, just adjacent to the posterior median septum, and contains axons arising from dorsal root ganglia T7 and below. The fasciculus cuneatus is located more laterally, between the fasciculus gracilis and the posterior horn of gray matter, and it contains axons from nerves in the dorsal root ganglia T6 and above. From the nucleii in the medulla, the axons of the secinary neurons cross to the contralateral side and progress to the posterior lateral nucleus of the thalamus where they synapse with neurons that project to the precentral gyrus.

Ascending Pathways in the Lateral Funiculus:

Lateral Spinothalamic - This tract carries sensations of pain and temperature from free nerve ending receptors throughout the body. Central processes of neurons, whose bodies are in the dorsal root ganglion, enter the cord at Lissauer's fasciculus, the white matter at the edge of the dorsal horn. From there they ascend the cord one or two spinal segments before entering the dorsal horn and synapsing with secondary neurons. These cross to the contralateral side through the white commisure and travel up the cord in the lateral spinothalamic tract located at the lateral aspect of the cord, just medial to the anterior spinocerebellar tract. As axons join the tract, they are added medially, so fibers relating to the lower body are in the lateral part of the tract. The secondary neurons ascend to several nuclei in the thalamus including the ventral posterior lateral nucleus (VPL) after giving off branches to the periaquiductal gray and reticular formation of the brain stem. These collaterals may play a role in pain transmission in the area.

Posterior Spinocerebellar and Cuneocerebellar - These tracts carry muscle position and movement information from muscle spindles and golgi tendon organs to the cerebellum. This tract never reaches the cerebrum and therefore the proprioception is unconscious. The posterior spinocerebellar tract is concerned with the lower half of the body, below C8, while the cueocerebellar tract is concerned with information above C8. From L3 to C8, primary neurons project into the posterior columns and synapse in a nucleus in the center gray matter called Clarke's column (which only exists in these segments). The secondary neurons send their axons laterally to the posterior spinocerebellar tract which ascends to the inferior cerebellar peduncle and into the cerebellum. Neurons entering the cord below the L3 level ascend in the posterior columns to L3, where they can go to Clarke's column. Primary neurons entering the cord higher than C8 enter the posterior column and synapse in the cuneate mucleus in the medulla. From there the secondary neurons continue rostrally as the cuneocerebellar tract, through the inferior penduncle and into the cerebellum.

Rostral Spinocerebellar and Anterior Spinocerebellar - These tracts carry postural information from muscle spindle and golgi tendon organs regarding an entire limb to the cerebellum. Primary neurons of the rostral spinocerebellar track have their cell bodies in the spinal root ganglia of lumbar and sacral nerves. They synapse at the base of the dorsal horn and the secondary neurons cross to the contralateral side of the cord and ascend the cord in the anterior spinocerebellar tract, passing

- 15 -

through the superior penduncle into the cerebellum. The rostral spinocerebellar tract is the upper limb equivalent of the anterior spinothalamic tract. It has only been investigated in cats, so its pathway in humans is inferred. The primary neurons synapse at the base of the dorsal horn and the secondary neurons stay ipsilateral and ascend the cord in the rostral spinocerebellar tract, entering the cerebellum through either the inferior or superion penduncle.

Ascending Pathways of the Anterior Funiculus

Anterior Spinothalamic – This tract carries sensations of poorly localized crude touch, tickling, itching, and sex. It is continuous with the lateral spinothalamic and the separation between the two is not clearly defined. The primary neurons are receptors in the hairless skin of the body that have their cell bodies in the spinal ganglia and project into the posterior horn. There they synapse with secondary neurons that cross to the contralateral side of the cord and form the anterior spinothalamic tract. In the medulla this tract merges with the lateral spinothalamic tract and branches extensively to the reticular formation and lateral reticular nucleus. It ascends to the VPL nucleus and posterior region of the thalamus where the neurons synapse with tertiary neurons that project to the precentral gyrus of the cerebral cortex.

Descending Pathways

Lateral Corticispinal and Anterior Corticospinal – The corticospinal tract is the major descending pathway extending from the cerebral cortex and affecting both motor neurons and sensory interneurons in the spinal cord. The neurons arise from the primary motor cortex as well as the cortical areas of the parietal and temporal lobes. The axons descend from the cortex to become the internal capsule then continue caudally forming the pyramids in the medulla. At the junction between the medulla and spinal cord most (75 – 90%) of the fibers cross to the contralateral side forming the decussation of the pyramids. The crossed fibers continue their descent in the lateral funiculus as the lateral sorticospinal tract while the uncrossed fibers continue in the anterior funiculus as the anterior corticospinal tract. The anterior corticospinal tract usually does not extend past the thoracic segments and the fibers decussate at the cord segment where they terminate. About half of the fibers synapse with interneurons at the base of the posterior horn to modify sensory input. The remaining half synapse with anterior horn motor neurons and adjacent interneurons. From there the anterior horn motor neurons terminate at neuromuscular junctions for voluntary muscle control.

Rubrospinal – This tract descends from the red nucleus in the midbrain, in the lateral funiculus of the cord, as far as the thoracic segments. It is important in controlling flexor tone in the limbs and serves as another connection of the cortex to the spinal cord through the inputs of the cerebral cortex and the cerebellum to the red nucleus. The tract runs closely with the lateral corticospinal tract. The fibers terminate on interneurons in the anterior gray horn which synapse with motor neurons.

Tectospinal – This tract begins at the superior colliculus of the midbrain, which is important for cisual-following and eye-centering reflexes and descends down under the periaquiductal gray, crossing the midline and forming the dorsal termental decussation. It continues caudally in the anterior funiculus as far as the cervical cord and the terminal fibers synapse with interneurons which synapse in turn with anterior horn motor neurons. The function of the tract is not well established, though it is thought to combine visial and auditory stimuli with postural reflex movements.

Reticulospinal Tracts – These two tracts arise from several layers in the brain stem reticular core and modify motor and sensory functions of the spinal cord. They can inhibit of fascilitale muscle activity and tone, influence respiration and circulation, and affect transmission on sensory impulses. The pontine reticulospinal tract originates at the pontine tegmentum and descends in the anterior funiculus, remaining uncrossed. The terminal fibers end on interneurons that project to both alpha motor neurons, affecting extrafusal muscle fibers, and gamma motor neurons, innervating intrafusal fibers of muscle spindles. The medullary reticulospinal tract arises from the medial 2/3 of the medulla and descends in the anterior funiculus, also remaining uncrossed. The terminal fibers go to interneurons that send their axons to both alpha and gamma motor neurons.

Vestibulospinal – This tract facilitales activity of extensor (antigravity) muscles providing basic posture. It arises from cells in the lateral vestibular nucleus in the medulla and descends ipsilaterally in the anterior funiculus. The vestibular nuclei all receive input from the vestibular organs of the inner ear and fromt he cerebellum. The tract gives off terminal fibers at each segment that synapse with interneurons , which project to anterior horn motor neurons.

Spinal Cord Injuries and Conditions

Complete injury: there is a complete loss of function below the level of the lesion, with no sensation or motor function in the S4-S5 dermatome segments, or the lowest sacral segment (adapted from ASIA).
Incomplete injury: there is a partial loss of sensory and/or motor function below the level of the lesion, to include the lowest sacral segment (adapted from ASIA).
Autonomic dysreflexia: response to a noxious stimulus, such as tight garments or distended bladder, in an individual with a lesion higher than T6. Symptoms include headache, profuse sweating, increased blood pressure and flushing. If removal of the stimulus does not resolve the symptoms, it is considered to be a medical emergency.
Orthostatic hypotension: fall in blood pressure associated with assuming upright posture due to blood rushing to the legs. It can be resolved by elevating the legs, or by reclining the patient.
Heterotopic ossification: calcification in the connective tissue surrounding a joint resulting in abnormal pathological bone formation. The result is pain, swelling and decreased range of motion.

Basal Ganglia Review

The basal ganglia form the major inputs to the ventral lateral nucleus of the thalamus, which in turn provides major inputs to area 6, comprised of the PMA and SMA, The basal ganglia is a collection of subcortical nuclei including the following:
- caudate nucleus and putamen (called the striatum)
- globus pallidus
- subthalamus
- substantia nigra

Spina bifida

The least severe type of spina bifida is termed spina bifida occulta. It is also the most prevalent. In this form, there is a cleft spine, however there is little or no damage to the nerves and spinal cord itself. Neurological function is generally intact, with the exception of possible neurogenic complications of the bowel and bladder.

Meningocele is the second most severe version of spina bifida, and refers to the condition in which the meninges protrude in a pouch from a vertebral gap. The spinal cord remains intact, however surgery is usually required to remove the sac. Occasionally motor or sensory deficits may exist, but meningocele is usually resolved following surgery.

Myelomeningocele is the most severe form of the disorder, and refers to a condition in which both the meninges and the spinal cord are pushed through a vertebral gap. The spinal cord and/or nerves below the lesion are usually damaged, resulting in sensory and motor deficits.

Respiratory Review

Inspiratory Values and Terms
- Inspiratory Reserve Volume (IRV)
    - Maximal inspired volume from end tidal inspiration
- Tidal Volume (Vt)
    - Volume inspired and expired with each normal breath
    - Minimum volume: 3 ml/kg
    - Normal volume: 6-7 ml/kg
- Inspiratory Capacity (IC)
    - Maximal volume inspired from resting expiratory level
    - Calculation: IRV + Vt

Expiratory Values and Terms
- Expiratory Reserve Volume (ERV)
    - Maximal expired volume from end-tidal inspiration
    - Normal: 25% of Vital Capacity
- Residual Volume (RV)
    - Volume remaining in lungs after maximal expiration
    - Normal adult: 1.0 to 2.4 Liters
- Functional Residual Capacity (FRC)
    - Volume remaining in lungs at resting expiratory level

Overall Lung Values and Terms
- Vital Capacity (VC)
    - Maximal volume expelled after maximal inspiration
- Total Lung Capacity (TLC)
    - Volume in lungs at end of maximal inspiration
    - Calculation: VC + RV
    - Normal adult: 4-6 Liters

CO = SV x HR
(Cardiac Output) = (Stroke Volume) x (Heart Rate)

$$EF = \frac{SV}{EDV} \times 100\%$$

(Ejection fracture) = (Stroke volume)

(End diastolic volume)

Breath Sounds

1. Friction rub- This is a harsh grating noise that may be audible as an adventitial breath sound when auscultating the lung fields. The sound is created when thickened, roughened, or irritated pleural membranes rub together as the lungs expand and contract.
2. Stridor- Continuous adventitious sound of inspiration associated with upper airway obstruction
3. Rales (crackles)- short explosive popping sounds due to alveoli suddenly opening.
4. Rhonchi – Coarse, low-pitched breath sounds heard in patients with chronic mucus in the airways.
5. Wheezes – Musical sound as air passes rapidly through narrowed bronchi.

Important Information

Acid/Base Balance	pH	Causes
Respiratory Alkalosis	Up	Alveolar hyperventilation
Respiratory Acidosis	Down	Alveolar hypoventilation
Metabolic Alkalosis	Up	(Steroids, or Vomiting)
Metabolic Acidosis	Down	(Diabetic, Uremic acidosis)

Chronic Bronchitis

COPD-Chronic Bronchitis/Emphysema-abnormal expiratory flow rates.
Signs and Symptoms
1. Smoking History
2. Cor pulmonale
3. Decreased expiratory flow rates
4. Crackles and wheezes
5. Hypoxemia

Emphysema
Signs and Symptoms
1. Barralled chest
2. Dyspnea
3. Cyanosis
4. Clubbing
5. Accessory muscles of ventilation

Important Information

Term	Obstructive Disease	Restrictive Disease
Total lung capacity	increases	decreases
Functional residual capacity	increases	decreases
Residual volume	increases	decreases
Vital capacity	decreases	decreases

Tuberculosis

Infectious respiratory process caused by tubercle bacilli.

Test-PPD-Purified Protein Derivative- Negative 0-4mm after 48 hours
Positive >10mm after 48 hrs.
Sputum + for *Mycobacterium tuberculosis* within 2-3 weeks of onset. Later (-) in the latent phase.
Drugs of choice in most cases Isoniazid and Rifampin.

Terminology:
Atelectasis - a collapsed or airless condition of the lung
Consolidation - the act of becoming solid. Ie. Solidification of the lungs due to pathological
engorgement of the lung tissues as occurs in acute pneumonia.
Egophony - a nasal sound, somewhat like the bleat of a goat, heard in auscultation of the chest wall
when the subject speaks in a normal tone. Often due to pleural effusion
Pleural effusion - fluid in the thoracic cavity between the visceral and parietal pleura
Bronchophony - Enhanced breath sounds auscultated over the bronchi
Whispered Pectoriloquy - distinct transmission of vocal sounds to the ear through the chest wall in
auscultation.

MET Review

"MET" is an abbreviation referring to a unit of "metabolic equivalent". One MET describes the energy it
takes to sit still. For the average adult, this is about one calorie per every 2.2 pounds of body weight
per hour someone who weighs 160 pounds would burn approximately 70 calories an hour while
sitting or sleeping.

MET Levels and Daily Activities	
	METs
Mild	
Playing the piano	2.3
Golf (with cart)	2.5
Dancing (ballroom)	2.9
Moderate	
Walking (3 mph)	3.3
Cycling (leisurely)	3.5
Calisthenics	4.0
Golf (no cart)	4.4
Walking	4.5
Vigorous	
Chopping wood	4.9
Tennis (doubles)	5.0
Skiing (water or downhill)	6.8
Climbing hills (no load)	6.9
Swimming	7.0
Walking (5 mph)	8.0

Rope skipping	12.0
Squash	12.1
Activities of daily living	
Lying quietly	1.0
Sitting; light activity	1.5
Walking from house to car or bus	2.5
Taking out trash	3.0
Walking the dog	3.0
Household tasks, moderate effort	3.5
Lifting items continuously	4.0
Raking lawn	4.0
Gardening (no lifting)	4.4
Mowing lawn (power mower)	4.5

Respiratory Conditions

Pulmonary Valve **Stenosis**

Causes:	*Symptoms:*	*Tests:*	*Treatment:*
Congenital	Fainting	Cardiac catheterization	Prostaglandins
Endocarditis	SOB	ECG	Dieuretics
Rheumatic Fever	Palpitations	Chest-Xray	Anti-arrhythmics
	Cyanosis	Echocardiogram	Blood thinners
	Poor weight gain		Valvuloplasty

ARDS- low oxygen levels caused by a build up of fluid in the lungs and inflammation of lung tissue.

Causes:	*Symptoms:*	*Treatment*:
Trauma	Low BP	Echocardiogram
Chemical inhalation	Rapid breathing	Auscultation
Pneumonia	SOB	Cyanosis
Septic shock	*Tests:*	Chest X-ray
	ABG	
	CBC	
	Cultures	

Mechanical Ventilation
Treat the underlying condition
Monitor the Patient for:
Pulmonary fibrosis
Multiple system organ failure
Ventilator associated pneumonia
Acidosis
Respiratory failure

Respiratory Acidosis- Build-up of Carbon Dioxide in the lungs that causes acid-base imbalances and the body becomes acidic.

Causes:	Symptoms:	Tests:	Treatment:
COPD	Chronic cough	CAT Scan	Mechanical
Airway obstruction	Wheezing	ABG	ventilation
Hypoventilation	SOB	Pulmonary Function	Bronchodilators
syndrome	Confusion	Test.	
Severe scoliosis	Fatigue		
Severe asthma			

Respiratory Alkalosis: CO_2 levels are reduced and pH is high.

Causes:	Symtpoms:	Tests:	Treatment:
Anxiety	Dizziness	ABG	Paper bag technique
Fever	Numbness	Chest X-ray	Increase carbon
Hyperventilation		Pulmonary function	dioxide levels
		tests	

RSV (Respiratory synctial virus) - spread by contact, virus can survive for various time periods on different surfaces.

Symptoms:	Tests:	Treatment:	Monitor the patient for:
Fever	ABG	Ribvirin	Pneumonia
SOB	Chest X-ray	Ventilator in severe	Respiratory failure
Cyanosis		cases	Otitis Media
Wheezing		IV fluids	
Nasal congestion		Bronchodilators	
Croupy cough			

Hyperventilation
Causes:
COPD
Panic Attacks
Stress
Ketoacidosis
Aspirin overdose
Anxiety

Apnea: no spontaneous breathing.
Causes:
Obstructive sleep apnea
Seizures
Cardiac Arrhythmias
Brain injury
Nervous system dysfunction
Drug overdose
Prematurity
Bronchospasm
Encephalitis
Choking

Lung surgery

Causes:
Cancer
Lung abscesses
Atelectasis
Emphysema
Pneumothorax
Tumors
Bronchiectasis

Pneumonia: viruses are the primary cause in young children; bacteria are the primary cause in adults. Bacteria: Streptococcus pneumoniae, Mycoplasma pneumoniae *pneumoniae* (pneumococcus).

Types of pneumonia:	Symptoms:	Tests:	Treatment:
Viral pneumonia	Fever	Chest X-ray	Antibiotics (if caused by a
Walking pneumonia	Headache	Pulmonary perfusion	bacterial infection)
Legionella pneumonia	Ribvirin	scan	Respiratory treatments
CMV pneumonia	SOB	CBC	Steroids
Aspiration pneumonia	Cough	Cultures of sputum	IV fluids
Atypical pneumonia	Chest pain	Presence of crackles	Vaccine treatments
Legionella pneumonia			

Pulmonary actinomycosis –bacteria infection of the lungs caused by (propionibacteria or actinomyces)

Causes:	Symptoms:	Tests:	Monitor patient for:
Microorganisms	Pleural effusions	CBC	Emphysema
	Facial lesions	Lung biopsy	Meningitis
	Chest pain	Thoracentesis	Osteomyelitis
	Cough	CT scan	
	Weight loss	Bronchoscopy	
	Fever		

Alveolar proteinosis: A build-up of a phospholipid in the lungs were carbon dioxide and oxygen are transferred.

Causes:	Symptoms:	Tests:	Treatment:
May be associated	Weight loss	Chest X-ray	Lung transplantation
with infection	Fatigue	Presence of crackles	Special lavage of the
Genetic disorder 30-	Cough	CT scan	lungs
50 yrs. Old	Fever	Bronchoscopy	
	SOB	ABG- low O2 levels	
		Pulmonary Function tests	

Pulmonary hypertension: elevated BP in the lung arteries

Causes:	Symptoms:	Tests:	Treatment:
May be genetically	Fainting	Pulmonary arteriogram	Manage symptoms
linked	Fatigue	Chest X-ray	Diuretics
More predominant	Chest Pain	ECG	Calcium channel blockers

| in women | SOB with activity
LE edema
Weakness | Pulmonary function tests
CT scan
Cardiac catheterization | Heart/Lung Transplant if
necessary |

Pulmonary arteriovenous fistulas: a congenital defect were lung arteries and veins form improperly, and a fistula is formed creating poor oxygenation of blood.

Symptoms:	*Tests:*	*Treatment:*
SOB with activity	CT Scan	Surgery
Presence of a murmur	Pulmonary arteriogram	Embolization
Cyanosis	Low O2 Saturation levels	
Clubbing	Elevated RBC's	
Paradoxical embolism		

Pulmonary aspergilloma: fungal infection of the lung cavities causing abscesses.

Cause:	*Symptoms:*	*Tests:*	*Treatment:*
Fungus *Aspergillus*	Wheezing	CT scan	Surgery
	SOB	Sputum culture	Antifungal medications
	Chest pain	Serum precipitans	
	Fever	Chest X-ray	
	Cough	Bronchoscopy	

Pulmonary edema: most commonly caused by Heart Failure, but may be due to lung disorders.

Symptoms:	*Tests:*	*Treatment:*
Restless behavior	Murmurs may be present	Diuretics
Anxiety	Echocardiogram	Oxygen
Wheezing	Presence of crackles	Treat the underlying cause
Poor speech	Low O2 Saturation levels	
SOB		
Sweating		
Pale skin		
Drowning sensation		

Idiopathic pulmonary fibrosis: Thickening of lung tissue in the lower aspects of the lungs.

Causes:	*Symptoms:*	*Tests:*
Response to an inflammatory agent	Cough	Pulmonary function tests
Found in people ages 50-70.	SOB	Lung biopsy
Linked to smoking	Chest pain	Rule out other connective tissue diseases
	Cyanosis	CT scan
	Clubbing	Chest X-ray
	Cyanosis	

Treatment:	*Monitor the patient for:*
Lung transplantation	Polycythemia
Corticosteroids	Pulmonary Htn.
Anti-inflammatory drugs	Respiratory failure
	Cor pulmonarle

Pulmonary emboli: Blood clot of the pulmonary vessels or blockage due to fat droplets, tumors or parasites.

Causes:	Symptoms:	
DVT- most common	SOB (rapid onset)	Dizziness
	Chest pain	Anxiety
	Decreased BP	Tachycardia
	Skin color changes	Labored breathing
	LE and pelvic pain	Cough
	Sweating	

Tests:	Treatment:	Monitor the patient for:
Doppler US	Placement of an IVC filter	Shock
Chest X-ray	Administer Oxygen	Pulmonary hypertension
Pulmonary angiogram	Surgery	Hemorrhage
Pulmonary perfusion test	Thrombolytic Therapy if	Palpitations
Plethysmography	clot detected	Heart failure
ABG		
Check O2 saturation		

Tuberculosis- infection caused by *Mycobaterium tuberculosis.*

Causes:	Symptoms:	Tests:
Due to airborne exposure	Fever	Thoracentesis
	Chest pain	Sputum cultures
	SOB	Presence of crackles
	Weight Loss	TB skin test
	Fatigue	Chest X-ray
	Wheezing	Bronchoscopy
	Phlegm production	

Treatment:
Generally about 6 months
Rifampin
Pyrazinamide
Isoniazid

Cytomegalovirus – can cause lung infections and is a herpes-type virus.

Causes:
More common in immunocompromised patients
Often associated with organ transplantation

Symptoms:	Tests:
Fever	CMV serology tests
SOB	ABG
Fatigue	Blood cultures
Loss of appetite	Bronchoscopy
Cough	
Joint pain	

Treatment:	Monitor the patient for:
Antiviral medications	Kidney dysfunction
Oxygen therapy	Infection

Decreased WBC levels

Relapses Viral pneumonia – inflammation of the lungs caused by viral infection.

Causes:	*Symptoms:*
Rhinovirus	Fatigue
Herpes simplex virus	Sore Throats
Influenza	Nausea
Adenovirus	Joint pain
Hantavirus	Headaches
CMV	Muscular pain
RSV	Cough
	SOB

Tests:	*Treatment:*
Bronchoscopy	Antiviral medications
Open Lung biopsy	IV fluids
Sputum cultures	
Viral blood tests	

Monitor the patient for:
Liver failure
Heart failure
Respiratory failure

Pneumothorax: a build-up of a gas in the pleural cavities.

Types:	*Symptoms:*
Traumatic pneumothorax	SOB
Tension pneumothorax	Tachycardia
Spontaneous pneumothorax	Hypotension
Secondary spontaneous pneumothorax	Anxiety
	Cyanosis
	Chest pain-sharp
	Fatigue

Tests:	*Treatment:*
ABG	Chest tube insertion
Chest X-ray	Administration of oxygen
Poor breath sounds	

Circulatory System

Functions

The circulatory system serves:
1. to conduct nutrients and oxygen to the tissues;
2. to remove waste materials by transporting nitrogenous compounds to the kidneys and carbon dioxide to the lungs;
3. to transport chemical messengers (hormones) to target organs and modulate and integrate the internal milieu of the body;
4. to transport agents which serve the body in allergic, immune, and infectious responses;
5. to initiate clotting and thereby prevent blood loss;
6. to maintain body temperature;
7. to produce, carry and contain blood;
8. to transfer body reserves, specifically mineral salts, to areas of need.

General Components and Structure

The circulatory system consists of the heart, blood vessels, blood and lymphatics. It is a network of tubular structures through which blood travels to and from all the parts of the body. In vertebrates this is a completely closed circuit system, as William Harvey (1628) once demonstrated. The heart is a modified, specialized, powerful pumping blood vessel. Arteries, eventually becoming arterioles, conduct blood to capillaries (essentially endothelial tubes), and venules, eventually becoming veins, return blood from the capillary bed to the heart.

Course of Circulation

Systemic Route

Arterial system. Blood is delivered by the pulmonary veins (two from each lung) to the left atrium, passes through the bicuspid (mitral) valve into the left ventricle and then is pumped into the ascending aorta; backflow here is prevented by the aortic semilunar valves. The aortic arch toward the right side gives rise to the brachiocephalic (innominate) artery which divides into the right subclavian and right common carotid arteries. Next, arising from the arch is the common carotid artery, then the left subclavian artery.

The subclavians supply the upper limbs. As the subclavian arteries leave the axilla (armpit) and enter the arm (brachium), they are called brachial arteries. Below the elbow these main trunk lines divide into ulnar and radial arteries, which supply the forearm and eventually form a set of arterial arches in the hand which give rise to common and proper digital arteries. The descending (dorsal) aorta continues along the posterior aspect of the thorax giving rise to the segmental intercostals arteries. After passage "through" (behind) the diaphragm it is called the abdominal aorta.

At the pelvic rim the abdominal aorta divides into the right and left common iliac arteries. These divide into the internal iliacs, which supply the pelvic organs, and the external iliacs, which supply the lower limb.

Venous system. Veins are frequently multiple and variations are common. They return blood originating in the capillaries of peripheral and distal body parts to the heart.

Hepatic Portal System: Blood draining the alimentary tract (intestines), pancreas, spleen and gall bladder does not return directly to the systemic circulation, but is relayed by the hepatic portal system of veins to and through the liver. In the liver, absorbed foodstuffs and wastes are processed. After processing, the liver returns the blood via hepatic veins to the inferior vena cava and from there to the heart.

Pulmonary Circuit: Blood is oxygenated and depleted of metabolic products such as carbon dioxide in the lungs.

Lymphatic Drainage: A network of lymphatic capillaries permeates the body tissues. Lymph is a fluid similar in composition to blood plasma, and tissue fluids not reabsorbed into blood capillaries are transported via the lymphatic system eventually to join the venous system at the junction of the left internal jugular and subclavian veins.

The Heart

The heart is a highly specialized blood vessel which pumps 72 times per minute and propels about 4,000 gallons (about 15,000 liters) of blood daily to the tissues. It is composed of:
> Endocardium (lining coat; epithelium)
> Myocardium (middle coat; cardiac muscle)
> Epicardium (external coat or visceral layer of pericardium; epithelium and mostly connective tissue)
> Impulse conducting system

*Cardiac Nerves***:** Modification of the intrinsic rhythmicity of the heart muscle is produced by cardiac nerves of the sympathetic and parasympathetic nervous system. Stimulation of the sympathetic system increases the rate and force of the heartbeat and dilates the coronary arteries. Stimulation of the parasympathetic (vagus nerve) reduces the rate and force of the heartbeat and constricts the coronary circulation. Visceral afferent (sensory) fibers from the heart end almost wholly in the first four segments of the thoracic spinal cord.

*Cardiac Cycle***:** Alternating contraction and relaxation is repeated about 75 times per minute; the duration of one cycle is about 0.8 second. Three phases succeed one another during the cycle:
> a) atrial systole: 0.1 second,
> b) ventricular systole: 0.3 second,
> c) diastole: 0.4 second

The actual period of rest for each chamber is 0.7 second for the atria and 0.5 second for the ventricles, so in spite of its activity, the heart is at rest longer than at work.

Blood: Blood is composed of cells (corpuscles) and a liquid intercellular ground substance called plasma. The average blood volume is 5 or 6 liters (7% of body weight). Plasma constitutes about 55% of blood volume, cellular elements about 45%.

Plasma: Over 90% of plasma is water; the balance is made up of plasma proteins and dissolved electrolytes, hormones, antibodies, nutrients, and waste products. Plasma is isotonic (0.85% sodium chloride). Plasma plays a vital role in respiration, circulation, coagulation, temperature regulation, buffer activities and overall fluid balance.

Cardiovascular Conditions

Cardiogenic Shock: heart is unable to meet the demands of the body. This can be caused by conduction system failure or heart muscle dysfunction.

Symptoms of Shock:
Rapid breathing
Rapid pulse
Anxiety
Nervousness
Thready pulse
Mottled skin color
Profuse sweating
Poor capilary refill

Tests:
Nuclear Scans
Electrocardiogram
Echocardiogram
Electrocardiogram
ABG
Chem-7
Chem-20
Electrolytes
Cardiac Enzymes

Treatment:
Amrinone
Norepinephrine
Dobutamine
IV fluids
PTCA
Extreme cases-pacemaker, IABP

Aortic insufficiency: Heart valve disease that prevents the aortic valve from closing completely. Backflow of blood into the left ventricle.

Causes:
Rheumatic fever
Congenital abnormalities
Endocarditis
Marfan's syndrome
Ankylosing spondylitis
Reiter's syndrome

Symptoms:
Fainting
Weakness
Bounding pulse
Chest pain on occasion
SOB
Fatigue

Tests:
Palpation
Increased pulse pressure and diastolic pressure
Pulmonary edema present
Auscultation
Left heart cathereterization
Aortica angiography
Dopper US

Treatment:
Digoxin
Dieuretics
Surgical aorta valve repair

Monitor patient for:
PE
Left-sided heart failure

Echocardiogram   Endocarditis

Aortic aneurysm: Expansion of the blood vessel wall often identified in the thoracic region.

Causes: *Symptoms:*
Htn   Possible back pain may be the only indicator
Marfan's syndrome
Syphilis
Atherosclerosis (most common)
Trauma

Tests: *Monitor patient for:*
Aortogram   Bleeding
Chest CT   Stroke
X-ray   Graft infection
Treatment: Irregular Heartbeats
Varies depending on location   Heart Attack
Stent
Circulatory arrest
Surgery

Hypovolemic shock: Poor blood volume prevents the heart from pumping enough blood to the body.

Causes:
Trauma
Diarrhea
Burns
GI Bleeding

Cardiogenic shock: Enough blood is available, however the heart is unable to move the blood in an effective manner.

Symptoms: *Tests:*
Anxiety   CBC
Weakness   Echocardiogram
Sweating   CT scan
Rapid pulse   Endoscopy with GI bleeding
Confusion   Swan-Ganz catheterization
Clammy skin   *Treatment:*
                                                    Increase fluids via IV
                                                    Avoid Hypothermia
                                                    Epinephrine
                                                    Norepinephrine
                                                    Dobutamine
                                                    Dopamine

Myocarditis: inflammation of the heart muscle.

Causes: *Symptoms:*   *Tests:*

Bacterial or Viral Infections
Polio, adenovirus, coxsackie virus

Leg edema
SOB
Viral symptoms
Joint Pain
Syncope
Heart attack (Pain)
Fever
Unable to lie flat
Irregular heart beats

Chest X-ray
Echocardiogram
ECG
WBC and RBC count
Blood cultures

Treatment:
Diuretics
Pacemaker
Antibiotics
Steroids

Monitor the patient for:
Pericarditis
Cardiomyopathy

Heart valve infection: endocarditis (inflammation), probable valvular heart disease. Can be caused by fungi or bacteria.

Symptoms:
Weakness
Fever
Murmur
SOB
Night sweats
Janeway lesions
Joint pain

Tests:
CBC
ESR
ECG
Blood cultures
Enlarged speen
Presence of splinter hemorrhages

Treatment:
IV antibiotics
Surgery may be indicated

Monitor the patient for:
Jaundice
Arrhythmias
CHF
Glomerulonephritis
Emboli

Pericarditis: Inflammation of the pericardium.

Causes:
Viral- coxsackie, adenovirus, influenza, rubella viruses
Bacterial (various microorganisms)
Fungi
Often associated with TB, Kidney failure, AIDS, and autoimmune disorders.
Surgery

Symptoms:
Dry cough
Pleuritis
Fever
Anxiety
Crackles
Pleural effusion
LE swelling
Chest pain
Unable to lie down flat

Tests:
Auscultation
MRI scan
CT scan
Echocardiogram (key test)
ESR
Chest x-ray
Blood cultures
CBC

Treatment:
NSAIDS
Pericardiocentesis

Monitor the patient for:
Constrictive pericarditis
A fib.

- 31 -

| Analgesics | Supraventricular tachycardia |
| Pericardiectomy | (SVT) |

Arrhythmias: Irregular heart beats and rhythms disorder

Types:	*Symptoms:*	*Tests:*
Bradycardia	SOB	Coronary angiography
Tachycardia	Fainting	ECG
Ventricular fibrillation	Palpitations	Echocardiogram
Ectopic heart beat	Dizziness	Holter monitor
Ventricular tachycardia	Chest pain	
Wolff-Parkinson-white	Irregular pulse	
syndrome		
Atrial fib.		
Sick sinus syndrome		
Sinus Tachycardia		
Sinus Bradycardia		

Treatment:	*Monitor the patient for:*
Defibrillation	Heart failure
Pacemaker	Stroke
Medications	Heart attack
	Ischemia

Arteriosclerosis: hardening of the arteries.

Causes:	*Symptoms:*	*Tests:*
Smoking	Claudication pain	Doppler US
Htn	Cold feet	Angiography
Kidney disease	Muscle acheness and pain in the	IVSU
CAD	legs	MRI test
Stroke	Hair loss on the legs	Poor ABI (Ankle brachial index)
	Numbness in the extremities	reading
	Weak distal pulse	

Treatment:	*Monitor the patient for:*
Analgesics	Arterial emboli
Vasodilation medications	Ulcers
Surgery if severe	Impotence
Ballon surgery	Gas gangreene
Stent placement	Infection of the lower
	extremities

Cardiomyopathy- poor hear pumping and weakness of the myocardium.

Causes:	*Types:*
Htn	Alcoholic cardiomyopathy- due to alcohol consumption
Heart attacks	Dilated cardiomyopathy-left ventricle enlargement
Viral infections	Hypertrophic cardiomyopathy-abnormal growth left ventricle
	Ischemic cardiomyopathy- weakness of the myocardium due to heart
	attacks.
	Peripartum cardiomyopathy- found in late pregnancy

- 32 -

Restrictive cardiomyopathy-limited filling of the heart due to inability to relax heart tissue.

Symptoms:	Tests:	Treatment:
Chest pain	ECG	Ace inhibitors
SOB	CBC	Dieuretics
Fatigue	Isoenzyme tests	Blood thinners
Ascites	Coronary Angigraphy	LVAD – Left Ventricular Assist
LE swelling	Chest X-ray	Device
Fainting	MRI	Digoxin
Poor Appetite	Auscultation	Vasodilators
Htn		
Palpitations		

Heart Sounds

S1- tricuspid and mitral valve close
S2- pulmonary and aortic valve close
S3- ventricular filling complete
S4-elevated atrial pressure (atrial kick)

Wave Review

ST segment:	ventricles depolarized
P wave:	atrial depolarization
PR segment:	AV node conduction
QRS complex:	ventricular depolarization
U wave:	hypokalemia creates a U wave
T wave:	ventricular repolarization

Other conditions

Congestive heart failure-CHF occurs when the heart is not able to meet the circulatory needs of the body and is characterized by decreased cardiac output, weakness and fatigue, shortness of breath and edema in the lower extremities.

Myocardial infarction-MI is caused by tissue death in the cardiac muscle resulting from lack of oxygenated blood in the arteries supplying the heart. Symptoms include radiating sub-sternal pain to the left arm, neck or jaw in addition to shortness of breath and nausea.

Deep venous thrombosis-DVT occurs when a clot or thrombus is formed in a vein, typically in the legs. If the clot travels through the bloodstream, it can trigger a cerebral vascular accident or pulmonary embolism. Signs include increased temperature or flushing in the involved extremity, as well as pain and edema.

Chronic obstructive pulmonary disease-COPD can include asthma, emphysema and chronic bronchitis, and is characterized by restrictive flow of air to and from the lungs. It is generally a progressive disorder and is often accompanied by anxiety.

Sternal and pacemaker precautions

Sternal precautions can vary in their specificity depending on the surgeon's preferences, however most physicians place restrictions on how much weight the patient can lift. This is usually five to ten pounds. Patients are instructed not to push or pull with force, and not to participate in activities that encourage broadening of the chest (i.e. aggressive horizontal abduction). After a pacemaker has been placed, the patient is instructed not to lift, push or pull as described above with the left upper extremity. Shoulder flexion and abduction are generally restricted to 90 degrees. The right upper extremity is usually not included in these precautions.

Patients recovering from heart surgery should be instructed on getting in and out of bed without using their arms forcefully. They should also be encouraged to work with their arms below shoulder height, and may benefit from extended handles to assist in brushing or washing their hair. Care should be taken during upper body dressing to ensure shoulder flexion is within allowable limits.

Rating of Perceived Exertion Scale

```
6 No exertion at all
7 Extremely light
8
9 Very light - (easy walking slowly at a comfortable pace)
10
11 Light
12
13 Somewhat hard (It is quite an effort; you feel tired but can continue)
14
15 Hard (heavy)
16
17 Very hard (very strenuous, and you are very fatigued)
18
19 Extremely hard (You can not continue for long at this pace)
20 Maximal exertion
```

Arrhythmias Review

Supraventricular Tachyarrhythmias

Atrial fibrillation – Abnormal QRS rhythm and poor P wave appearance. (>300bpm.)
Sinus Tachycardia- Elevated ventricular rhythum/rate.
Paroxysmal atrial tachycardia- Abnormal P wave, Normal QRS complex
Atrial flutter- Irregular P Wave development. (250-350 bpm.)
Paroxysmal supraventricular tachycardia- Elevated bpm (160-250)
Multifocal atrial tachycardia- bpm (>105). Various P wave appearances.

Ventricular Tachyarrhythmias

Ventricular Tachycardia- Presence of 3 or greater PVC's (150-200bpm), possible abrupt onset. Possibly due to an ischemic ventricle. No P waves present.

(PVC)- Premature Ventricular Contraction- In many cases no P wave followed by a large QRS complex that is premature, followed by a compensatory pause.

Ventricular fibrillation- Completely abnormal ventricular rate and rhythum requiring emergency innervention. No effective cardiac output.

Bradyarrhythmias

AV block (primary, secondary (I,II) Tertiary
Primary- >.02 PR interval
Secondary (Mobitz I) – PR interval Increase
Secondary (Mobitz II) – PR interval (no change)
Tertiary- most severe, No signal between ventricles and atria noted on ECG. Probable use of Atrophine indicated. Pacemaker required.

Right Bundle Branch Block (RBBB)/Left Bundle Branch Block (LBBB)

Sinus Bradycardia- <60 bpm, with presence of a standard P wave.

Cardiac Failure Review

Right Sided Heart Failure
A. Right Upper Quadrant Pain
B. Right Ventricular heave
C. Tricuspid Murmur
D. Weight gain
E. Nausea
F. Elevated Right Atrial pressure
G. Elevated Central Venous pressure
H. Peripheral edema
I. Ascites
J. Anorexia
K. Hepatomegaly

Left Sided Heart Failure
A. Left Ventricular Heave
B. Confusion
C. Paroxysmal noturnal dyspnea
D. DOE
E. Fatigue
F. S_3 gallop
G. Crackles
H. Tachycardia
I. Cough
J. Mitral Murmur
K. Diaphoresis
L. Orthopnea

Endocrine Review

Hypothyroidism: Poor production of thyroid hormone:
Primary- Thyroid cannot meet the demands of the pituitary gland.
Secondary- No stimulation of the thyroid by the pituitary gland.

Causes:
Surgical thyroid removal
Irradiation
Congenital defects
Hashimoto's thyroiditis (key)

Symptoms:
Constipation
Weight gain
Weakness
Fatigue
Poor taste
Depression

Hoarse vocal sounds
Joint pain
Muscle weakness
Poor speech
Color changes

Tests:
Decreased BP and HR
Chest X-ray
Elevated liver enzymes,
prolactin, and cholesterol
Decreased T4 levels and serum
sodium levels
Presence of anemia
Low temperature
Poor reflexes

Treatment:
Increase thyroid hormone levels
Levothyroxine

Monitor the patient for:
Hyperthyroidism symptoms
following treatment
Heart disease
Miscarriage
Myxedema coma if untreated

Hyperthyroidism: excessive production of thyroid hormone.

Causes:
Iodine overdose
Thyroid hormone overdose
Graves' disease (key)
Tumors affecting the reproductive system

Symptoms:
Skin color changes
Weight loss
Anxiety
Possible goiter
Nausea
Sweating

Exophthalmos
Diarrhea
Hair loss
Elevated BP
Fatigue

Tests:
Elevated Systolic pressure noted
T3/T4 (free) levels increased
TSH levels reduced

Treatment:
Radioactive iodine
Surgery
Beta-blockers
Antithyroid drugs

Congenital adrenal hyperplasia: Excessive production of androgen and low levels of aldosterone and cortisol. (Geneticially inherited disorder). Different forms of this disorder that affect males and females differently.

Causes: Adrenal gland enzyme deficit causes cortisol and aldosterone to not be produced. Causing male sex characteristics to be expressed prematurely in boys and found in girls.

Symptoms:
Boys:
Small testes development

Tests:
Salt levels
Low levels of cotisol

Treatment:
Reconstructive surgery
Hydrocoristone

Enlarged penis development
Strong musculature appearance
Girls:
Abnormal hair growth
Low toned voice
Abnormal genitalia
Lack of menstruation

Low levels of aldosterone
Increased 17-OH progesterone
Increased 17-ketosteroids in
urine

Dexamethasone

Primary/Secondary Hyperaldosteronism
Primary Hyperaldosteronism: problem within the adrenal gland causing excessive production of aldosterone.
Secondary Hyperaldosteronism: problem found elsewhere causing excessive production of aldosterone.
Causes:
Primary:
Tumor affecting the adrenal gland
Possibly due to HBP

Secondary:
Nephrotic syndrome
Heart failure
Cirrhosis
Htn

Symptoms:
Paralysis
Fatigue
Numbness sensations
Htn
Weakness

Tests:
Increased urinary aldosterone
Abnormal ECG readings
Decreased potassium levels
Decreased renin levels

Treatment:
Primary: Surgery
Secondary: Diet/Drugs

Cushing's syndrome: Abnormal production of ACTH which in turn causes elevated cortisol levels.
Causes:
Corticosteroids prolonged use
Tumors

Symptoms:
Muscle weakness
Central obesity distribution
Back pain
Thirst
Skin color changes
Bone and joint pain

Htn
Headaches
Frequent urination
Moon face
Weight gain
Acne

Tests:
Dexamethasone suppression test
Cortisol level check
MRI- check for tumors

Treatment:
Surgery to remove tumor
Monitor corticosteroid levels

Monitor the patient for:
Kidney stones
Htn
Bone fractures
DM
Infections

Diabetic ketoacidosis: increased levels of ketones due to a lack of glucose.
Causes: Insufficient insulin causing ketone production which end up in the urine. More common in type I vs. type 2 DM.
Symptoms:
Low BP

Tests:
Elevated glucose levels

Abdominal pain
Headaches
Rapid breathing
Loss of appetite
Nausea
Fruit breath smell
Mental deficits

Increased amylase and potassium levels
Ketones in urine
Check BP

Treatment:
Insulin
IV fluids

Monitor the patient for:
Renal failure
MI
Coma
T3/T4 Review
Both are stimulated by TSH release from the Pituitary gland

T4 control basal metabolic rate
T4 becomes T3 within cells. (T3) Active form.
T3 radioimmunoassay- Check T3 levels
Hyperthyroidism- T3 increased, T4 normal- (in many cases)

Medications that increase levels of T4:
Methadone
Oral contraceptives
Estrogen
Cloffibrate

Medications that decrease levels of T4:
Lithium
Propranolol
Interferon alpha
Anabolic steroids
Methiamazole

Lymphocytic thyroiditis: Hyperthyroidism leading to hypothyroidism and then normal levels.
Causes: Lymphocytes permeate the thyroid gland causing hyperthyroidism initially.

Symptoms:
Fatigue
Menstrual changes
Weight loss
Poor temperature tolerance
Muscle weakness
Hyperthyroidism symptoms

Tests:
T3/T4 increased
Increased HR
Lymphocyte concentration noted with biopsy

Treatment:
Varies depending on symptoms. (Beta blockers may be used.)

Monitor the patient for:
Autoimmune thyroditis
Hashimoto's thyroiditis
Goiter
Stuma lymphomatosoma

Graves' disease: most commonly linked to hyperthyroidism, and is an autoimmune disease. Exophthalmos may be noted (protruding eyeballs). Excessive production of thyroid hormones.

Symptoms:
Elevated appetite
Anxiety
Menstrual changes
Fatigue
Poor temperature tolerance
Diplopia
Exophthalmos

Tests:
Elevated HR
Increased T3/T4 levels
Serum TSH levels are decreased
Goiter

Treatment:

Monitor the patient for:

- 38 -

Beta-blockers
Surgery
Prednisone
Radioactive iodine

Fatigue
CHF
Depression
Hypothyroidism (over-correction)

Type I diabetes (Juvenile onset diabetes)

Causes: Poor insulin production from the beta cells of the pancreas. Excessive levels of glucose in the blood stream that cannot be used due to the lack of insulin. Moreover, the patient continues to experience hunger, due to the cells not getting the fuel that they need. After 7-10 years the beta cells are completely destroyed in many cases.

Symptoms:
Weight loss
Vomiting
Nausea
Abdominal pain
Frequent urination
Elevated thirst

Tests:
Fasting glucose test
Insulin test
Urine analysis

Treatment:
Insulin
Relieve the diabetic ketoacidosis symptoms
Foot ulcer prevention

Monitor for infection:
Monitor for hypoglycemia conditions if type I is over-corrected.
Glucagon may need to be administered if hypoglycemia conditions are severe.
Monitor the patient for ketone build-up if type I untreated.
Get the eyes checked- once a year

Type II diabetes

Causes: The body does not respond appropriately to the insulin that is present. Insulin resistance is present in Type II diabetes. Results in hyperglycemia.

Risk factors for Type II Diabetes:
Obesity
Limited exercise individuals
Race-Minorities have a higher distribution
Elevated Cholesterol levels
Htn

Symptoms:
Blurred vision
Fatigue
Elevated appetite
Frequent urination
Thirst
Note: A person may have Type II and be symptom free.

Tests:
Random blood glucose test.
Oral glucose tolerance test
Fasting glucose test.

Treatment:
Tlazamide
Glimepiride
Control diet
Increase exercise levels
Repaglidine/Nateglinide

Glycosylated hemoglobin
BUN/ECG
Frequent blood sugar testing
Acarbose
Diabetic Ulcer prevention

Monitor the patient for:
Neuropathy
CAD
Increased cholesterol
Retinopathy
PVD
Htn

General Risk Factors for diabetes
- Bad diet
- Htn
- Weight distribution around the waist/overweight.
- Certain minority groups
- History of diabetes in your family
- Poor exercise program
- Elevated triglyceride levels

Hypoglycemia
(Low blood sugar)

Symptoms: | *Treatment:*

Feel weak and dizzy   Carbohydrates that can be absorbed quickly
May appear pale   (Such as a hard candy or orange juice)
Become less responsive   OT treatment should be postponed until the patient's blood sugars are
Suddenly seem confused   back to the normal levels.

Hyperglycemia
(Elevated blood sugar)
Symptoms:

Ketoacidosis   Neurological abnormalities
Sudden, severe thirst   Acetone breath
Weak pulse

Treatment:
Ketoacidosis is a medical emergency and EMS should be called immediately. The patient should be made comfortable until the response team arrives.

Pharmacology Review

Drug Nomenclature

1. Generic name: ex. - acetominophen
2. Trade name: ex. - TYLENOL, PANADOL

Routes of Drug Entry

Enteral
1. ORAL – easiest, safe, have 1st pass effect, large surface area for absoption, some medications irritate the GI, some medications may be degraded by the stomach.
2. SUB-LINGUAL – absorption through the oral mucosa with no 1st pass effect.
3. RECTAL- normally no 1st pass effect, usually used if patients are vomiting

Parenteral
1. INHALATION – absorbed in the lungs, quick action, may cause inflammation in the lungs.
2. INJECTION (types):

A. Intra-muscular – easy access, may treat muscle or prolonged release into circulation.
B. Subcutaneous – Injection just below the skin, causes a localized response. TB skin test.
C. Intra-arterial – used most commonly in chemotherapy also diagnostic procedures, drug introduced directly into the artery
D. Intravenous – can use an IV line, useful in emergencies, side effects appear quickly
E. Intrathecal – used with narcotic analgesics and local anesthetics. Drugs can reach the CNS and by-pass the blood brain barrier.

Parasympathetic Action	Sympathetic Action
Discrete Response	Diffuse Response
Cranial/ Sacral origination	thoraco-lumbar origination
Presynaptic neurons release Ach	Presynaptic neurons – Ach
Postsynaptic neurons release Ach	Postsynaptic neurons –NE
Conserves Fuel, maintains GI	Fight or Flight Response

Pharmacology Review Chart

Drug Suffix	Example	Action
-azepam	Diazepam	Benzodiazepine
-azine	Chlorpromazine	Phenothiazine
-azole	Ketoconazole	Anti-fungal
-barbital	Secobarbital	Barbiturate
-cillin	Methicillin	Penicillin
-cycline	Tetracycline	Antibiotic
-ipramine	Amitriptyline	Tricyclic Anti-depressant
-navir	Saquinavir	Protease Inhibitor
-olol	Timolol	Beta Antagonist
-oxin	Digoxin	Cardiac glycoside
-phylline	Theophylline	Methylxanthine
-pril	Enalapril	ACE Inhibitor
-terol	Albuterol	Beta 2 Agonist
-tidine	Ranitidine	H_2 Antagonist
-trophin	Somatotrophin	Pituitary Hormone
-zosin	Doxazosin	Alpha 1 Antagonist

Cardiovascular Pharmacology

Antiarrhythmics (Na+ channel blockers) (Class I)

Class IA
Procainamide
Disopyramide
Amiodarone
Quinidine
Class IB
Mexiletine

- 41 -

Lidocaine
Tocainide

Class IC
Flecainide
Encainide
Propafenone
Antiarrhythmics (Beta blockers) (Class II)
Metroprolol
Atenolol
Propranolol
Timolol
Esmolol

Antiarrhythmics (K+Channel blockers) (ClassIII)
Sotaolol
Amiodarone
Bretylium
Ibutilide

Antiarrhythmics (Ca2+ channel blockers) (Class IV)
Diltiazem
Verapamil

Calcium Channel Blockers:
Verapamil
Diltiazem
Nifedipine

Cardiac glycosides:
Digoxin
Dieuretics:
Loop Dieuretics
Hydrocholorothiazide

Sympathoplegics:
Beta blockers
Clonidine
Reserpine
Guanethidine
Prazosin

ACE Inhibitors:
Lisinopril
Enalapril
Captopril

K+ Sparing Dieuretics:
Spironolactone
Triamterene
Amiloride

CNS Pharmacology
Sympathomimetics:
Dopamine
Dobutamine
Epinephrine
Norephinephrine
Isoproterenol

Cholinomimetics:
Carbachol
Neostigmine
Pyridostigmine
Echothiophate
Bethanechol

Cholinoreceptor blockers:
Hexamethonium-Nicotinic blocker
Atropine-Muscarinic blocker

Beta blockers:
Atenolol
Nadolol
Propranolol

Metoprolol
Pindolol
Labetalol

Tricyclic Antidepressants:
Doxepine
Imipramine
Amitriptyline
Nortriptyline
Amitriptyline

Parkinson's Treatment:
L-dopa
Amantadine
Bromocriptine

Benzodiazepindes:
Iorazepam
Triazolam
Oxazepam
Diazepam

Opiod Analgesics:
Heroin
Methadone
Morphine
Codeine
Dextromethorphan
Meperidine

MAO Inhibitors:
Tranylcypromine
Phenelzine

Seroton specific Re-uptake inhibitors:
Paroxetine
Sertraline
Fluoxetine
Citalopram

Epilepsy Treatment:
Valproic acid
Phenobarbital
Benzodiazepines
Gabapentin
Ethosuximide
Carbamazepine

Barbiturates:
Pentobarbital
Thiopental
Phenobarbital
Secobarbital

IV Anethestics:
Midazolam
Ketamine
Morphine
Fentanyl
Propofol
Thiopental

Local Anesthetics:
Tetracaine
Procaine
Lidocaine

Neuroleptics (Antipsychotic drugs)
Chlorpromazine
Thioridazine
Clozapine
Fluphenazine
Haloperidol

Alpha 1 Selective blockers:
Terazosin
Prazosin
Doxazosin
Alpha 2 Selective blockers:
Yohimbine

Glaucoma Treatment:

Prostaglandins
Dieuretics
Alpha agonists
Beta Blockers
Cholinomimetics

Cancer Treatment Drugs:

Etoposide

Carmustine

Nitrosoureas

Throbolytics:

Cisplatin

Urokinase

Doxorubicin

Anistreplase

Incristine

Streptokinase

Paclitaxel

Alteplase

Methotrexate

5 – fluorouracil

6 – mercaptopurine

Lomustine

Busulfan

Cox 2 Inhibitors:

Rofecoxib

Naproxen

Celecoxib

Indomethacin

Ibuprofen

Diabetic Treatment:

Insulin- Key

Sulfonylureas:

Chlorpropamide

Metformin

Tolbutamide
Glyburide

Glitazones:

Asthma Treatment:

Rosiglitazone

Corticosteroids:

Troglitazone

Prednisone

Pioglitazone

Beclomethasone

Antileukotrienes:

Beta 2 agonists:

Zafirlukast

Salmeterol

Zileuton

Albuterol

Nonselective Beta agonists:

Muscarinic agonists:

Isoproterenolol

Ipratropium

H₂ blockers:

Tetracyclines:

Famotidine

Tetracycline

Nizatidine

Doxycycline

Cimetidine

Minocycline

RanitidineAnti-Microbial Drugs

Demeclocycline

Macrolides:
Carithormycin
Erythromycin
Azithromycin
Aminoglycosides:
Amikacin
Gentamicin
Neomycin
Tobramycin
Streptomycin

Protein Synthesis Inhibitors:
Chloramphenicol
Aminoglycosides
Tetracyclines

TB Medications:
Isoniazid
Rifampin
Ethambutol
Pyrazinamide
Ethambutol

Fluoroquinolones:
Ciprofloxacin
Sparfloxacin
Enaxacin
Nalidixic acid
Norfloxacin
Mortifloxacin

Sulfonamides:
Sulfadiazine
Sulfisoxazole
Sulfamethoxazole
Malaria Treatment:
Chlorquine
Quinine
Mefloquine

Additional Mentionable Anti-viral Drugs:
Acyclovir
Amatadine
Ribavirin
Zanamivir
Ganciclovir

HIV Treatment:
Zidovudine (AZT)
Nevirapine
Didanosine

Protease Inhibitors-(HIV)
Saquinavir
Retinonavir   Nelfinavir

Controlled Substance Categories

Schedule I	Highest potential abuse, used mostly for research. (heroin, peyote, marijuana)
Schedule II	High potential abuse, but used for therapeutic purposes (opioids, amphetamines and barbiturates)
Schedule III	Mild to moderate physical dependence or strong psychological dependence on both. (opioids such as codeine, hydrocodone that are combined with other non-opoid drugs)
Schedule IV	Limited potential for abuse and physical and/or psychological dependence (benzodiazepines, and some low potency opioids)
Schedule V	Lowest abuse potential of controlled substances. Used in cough medications and anti-diarrheal preps.

Nutrition

Six Key Nutrients

1. Water
2. Protein
3. Minerals
4. Vitamins
5. Carbohydrates
6. Fats

Water

1. Normal production of water in a human is around 2500-2700 ml per day.
2. The average adult is composed of about 55-60% water.
3. More water is required for children and during warm weather.
4. Water acts as the body's solvent.
5. Water can be found in intra and extra cellular tissues.
6. Adults should take in 2-3 L of fluid over the course of a normal day.
7. Monitor following burns, diarrhea, and hemorrhage.

Protein

1. Proteins are made up of amino acids.
2. Amino Acids can be broken down into essential and non-essential amino acids. At least 9 amino acids must be found in your diet and cannot be manufactured by your own body.
3. There are three types of proteins: Complete, Incomplete, and Complementary.
4. Complete proteins are found in meats, cheese and poultry. These contain all 8 essential amino acids.
5. Incomplete proteins are found in plants, nuts, grains and legumes
6. Complimentary proteins- foods that have to be combined to offer a complete protein presentation.
7. Digestion process of chymotrypsin, trypsin, carboxypeptidase, and pepsin act upon proteins.
8. Proteins help in the production of antibodies and tissue healing.
9. Proteins become an energy source if carbs/fat are not available.
10. Marasmus-starvation
11. Recommend 15% caloric intake to be protein.
12. Uric acid, Nitrogen, and Hydrogen are all byproducts of protein breakdown.
13. Amino acids are incorporated into various structural and functional proteins, including enzymes.
14. A starving person has a negative nitrogen balance, a growing child or pregnant woman has a positive nitrogen balance.

Minerals

1. Minerals help maintain the function of the various acids and bases in the body.
2. About 75% of the minerals are found in bones and teeth as calcium and phosphorus.
3. Minerals may function as catalyst for cell reactions.
4. Minerals help create compounds in some cases.
5. Magnesium, Calcium, Phosphorus, Sodium and Potassium are all considered minerals

6. Minerals are usually incorporated into organic molecules, although some occur in inorganic compounds or as free ions.
7. Homeostatic mechanics regulate mineral concentration in the body.
8. Minerals are responsible for about 4% of body weight.
9. Minerals are found in all types of tissue.
10. Minerals do not create energy in the body.
11. Calcium and Phosphorus are key minerals in body development and maintenance.
12. Sodium and Potassium help trigger cell reaction potentials.
13. Minerals are found primarily in unprocessed foods.

Major Minerals:

Calcium (Ca)
Sources: Milk, Cheese, Broccoli, Turnips
Function: Bones, Clotting, Cell wall integrity, Conduction of Nerve Impulses
Disorders: Deficient Clotting, Poor Bone Structure- Osteoporosis, Limited cell integrity.

Chlorine (Cl)
Sources: Salt
Function: Helps produce acid-base relationships that are balanced, helps with osmotic pressures and the production of hydrochloric acid, helps regulate pH.
Disorders: Excessive water loss may cause low levels of chlorine in the body.

Magnesium (Mg)
Sources: Leafy Vegetables, Whole grains, Legumes, Milk
Function: Bones, Teeth, Function as enzymes, Nerve conduction, functions in the production of ATP
Disorders: Nervous system dysfunction

Phosphorus (P)
Sources: Egg Yolk, Whole grains, Meat, Milk
Function: Helps with calcification, Maintains acid-base relationship, Works as an enzyme, occurs in the phospholipids of cell membranes
Disorders: Rickets, poor bone structure

Potassium (K)
Sources: Fruits, Whole grains, Fish and Poultry
Function: Nervous system conduction, acid-base relationship, regulation of pH
Disorders: Nausea, Weakness of muscles

Sodium (Na)
Sources: Salt, Fish, Poultry, Milk
Function: Acid-base relationship, Nerve system conduction, Uptake of glucose
Disorders: Nausea, weakness, Muscle spasms/cramping

Sulfur (S)
Sources: Egg, Cheese, Nuts, Meat
Function: Aids with B vitamin function and helps develop with development of connective tissue, found in Insulin, Biotin, and mucopolysaccharides
Disorders: None applicable.

Vitamins

1. Fat- Soluble vs. Water Soluble Vitamins
2. Fat Soluble- Vitamin A, D, E, K
3. Water Soluble – Vitamin C, B1, B2, B6, B12, Folic Acid and Niacin

Water Soluble Vitamins:
Vitamin C – Ascorbic Acid
Sources: Citrus, Strawberries, Potatoes, Tomatoes
Function: Helps with uptake of iron, and cell membranes, closely related chemically to monosaccharides
Disorders: Scurvy, Anemia, Pronounced bruising of tissue

Vitamin B1- Thiamine
Sources: Legumes, Wheat germ, Pork
Function: Helps with muscle and nerve function, active in the synthesis of essential sugars
Disorders: Anorexia, nerve dysfunction, Beriberi

Vitamin B2- Riboflavin
Sources: Enriched breads, Milk, Meats, Greens
Function: Lip color, metabolic process of nutrients, eyes, can function as a coenzyme
Disorders: Weight loss, eye dysfunction, and lips may become inflamed.

Vitamin B6 - Pyridoxine
Sources: Red Meats
Function: Hemoglobin production, synthesis of proteins
Disorders: CNS disorders, kidney stones, and nausea

Vitamin B12 – Cobalamin
Sources: **Animals products only**
Function: RBC production, protein breakdown
Disorders: Pernicious anemia

Folic Acid - Folacin
Sources: Most foods.
Function: RBC production and protein breakdown, coenzyme in the synthesis of DNA
Disorders: Anemia, Stomatitis

Niacin – Nicotinic Acid
Sources: Meats, Peanut Butter
Function: Growth, Nervous System and Digestive System
Disorders: Pellagra, Dermatitis

Fat Soluble Vitamins:
Vitamin A – Retinol
Sources: Whole milk, Fish, Leafy Vegetables and Yellow Vegetables
Function: Vision, Skin, Teeth, - stored in the Liver
Disorders: Poor Vision, Xerophthalmia, Bad Skin

Vitamin D – Calciferol
Sources: Milk, Fish oils
Function: Bones. Also synthesized in the skin.
Disorders: Teeth, Bad bone structure, Rickets

Vitamin E – Tocopherol
Sources: Leafy Vegetables, Wheat germ
Function: Antioxidant, Stabilizes RBC's, stored in muscles and adipose tissue.
Disorders: Anemia, RBC's are broken down

Vitamin K – Menadione
Sources: Pork liver, Leafy Vegetables
Function: Helps with prothrombin for blood clotting
Disorders: Hemorrhagic conditions

Carbohydrates

1. Three types of carbohydrates: polysaccharides, disaccharides, monosaccharides.
2. Polysaccharides- Glycogen, dietary fiber, and starch found in cereal, rice, corn and pasta.
3. Disaccharides- (double sugars) – maltose, lactose, sucrose, found in molasses, table sugar
4. Monosaccharides – (simple sugars) - Fructose, glucose, galactose found in fruit and honey
5. Energy is released from glucose by oxidation.
6. If inadequate amounts of glucose are available, amino acids may be converted to glucose.
7. Carbohydrates provide energy and help in the breakdown of fat.
8. Carbohydrates can only be used the form of simple sugars by the body.
9. Primary processing and uptake of carbohydrates occurs in the small intestine by the enzymes maltase, sucrase, and lactase.
10. Glucose is the simple sugar used by the CNS and glucose can be stored as glycogen (polysaccharide) until being used later.
11. High levels of carbohydrates can lead to weight gain, and poor nutritional status.
12. Studies indicate that approximately 55% of an adults intake is carbohydrates.
13. Carbohydrates are absorbed as monosaccharides.
14. Dietary fiber can be broken down into soluble and insoluble dietary fiber.
15. Glucose is regulated by Insulin and Glucagon (horomone).
16. Educate patients to reduce simple sugars and encourage patients to eat more complex carbohydrates.

Fats

1. Excessive fats can lead to weight gain, stroke, and heart disease.
2. There are two primary types of fat: saturated fats and unsaturated fats.
3. Saturated fats- completely maximized number of Hydrogen present. Examples: eggs, chocolate, dairy, coconut oil, meats, usually solid at room temperature.
4. Unsaturated fats- usually liquid at room temperature, do not have maximum number of Hydrogen atoms present. Examples: soybean and corn oil.
5. Fats provide insulation to the body.
6. Linoleic acid is an essential fatty acid.
7. Cholesterol is obtained in foods of animal origin only.

8. Fats help with the transportation of fat soluable vitamins.
9. Fats act as an energy source when carbohydrates are unavailable.
10. Fats help create linoleic acid which is an essential component not created in the human body.
11. Primary fat breakdown occurs in the small intestine, however, some is performed in the stomach by gastric lipase.
12. Fats can also be classified as visible or invisible.
13. Visible fats: Shortening, Meats, Margarine, Butter
14. Invisible fats: Cheese, Milk, Avocado
15. Recommend to your patients total intake of fat to be less than 30% of caloric intake.
16. Cholesterol is a fatty type complex and is found in healthy adults.
17. Cholesterol is divided into (HDL) and (LDL) cholesterol.
18. HDL- High density lipoprotein
19. LDL- Low density lipoprotein
20. High Cholesterol is noted as above 240mg/dl
21. Borderline – 200-240 mg/dl
22. <200 mg/dl Recommended
23. Recommend polyunsaturated fats to lower cholesterol levels to your patients.

Behavioral & Mental Health Review
Behavioral Science Developmental Milestones

One month
Fine Motor-Holds both hands in fists. Grasps object with palm reflexively.
Gross Motor-Moves extremities symmetrically. Drops head forward if held sitting. Lifts and turns head side to side when in prone.
Language-Responds to sound with startle. Responds to voice with decreased activity. Turns to localize, usually finds face or object and brightens.
Social/Play-Stares at brightly colored or patterned objects. Regards toys only when in front of eyes. Follows dangling toy to midline and vertically.

Two months
Fine Motor-Holds ring placed in hand briefly. Brings hand to mouth. Looks at hands (3 months). Holds hands open instead of clenched and brings to midline (3 months).
Gross Motor- Lifts head 45 degrees in prone position. Rolls stomach to back (2-4) months. Holds head erect in sitting position with some bobbing.
Language-Cries differently when hungry, uncomfortable or bored. Coos. Smiles when some talks. Responds to loud noises and alerts to familiar voices.
Social/Play-Follows moving person with eyes. Follows dangling toy past midline (3 months).

Four months
Fine Motor-Reaches for and grasps toy (eye-hand coordination at 5 months).
Gross Motor-Supports head when pulled to sit. Holds head steady when sitting. Sits with mid-to-lower truck support. Holds head 90 degrees when prone. Pushes up on arms and looks directly ahead. Rolls stomach to back.
Language-Laughs out loud. Squeals.
Social/Play-Initiates smile. Smiles and talks to self in mirror, pats image when close to mirror. Takes toy to mouth while on back.

- 51 -

Six months
Fine Motor-Transfers toy hand to hand. Uses raking grasp or small object. Holds 1-inch cube with opposed grasp. Reaches for and secures toy with either hand, supine or sitting. Uses toys to make noise by banging and shaking.
Gross Motor-Rolls stomach to back and back to stomach. Sits briefly leaning on hands (tripod position). Bears weight on feet and bounces when standing.
Language-Makes tongue/lip sounds (raspberries, clicks, smacks).
Social/Play-Grasps feet when lying on back. Enjoys vigorous frolic play. Notices mother especially; conscious of strangers.

Nine months
Fine Motor-Takes objects out of open container. Holds bottle. Feeds self-cracker. Uses pincer grasp on small objects.
Gross Motor-Sits erect well. Gets from lying to sitting. Creeps/crawls. Pulls self to full standing position. Cruises
Language-Babbles with repeated consonant-vowel sounds. Imitates syllables. Responds to name.
Social/Play-Plays peek-a-cake and waves bye-bye. Looks for hidden or dropped toy.

Twelve months
Fine motor-Holds cup to drink. Releases object purposefully. Uses pincer grasp well. Imitates actions/uses of objects
Gross Motor-Cruises, walks independently or with one hand held (9-12 months). Crawls on all fours. Lets self down from furniture with control. Stands alone at least momentarily.
Language-Follows simple commands. Jabbers with sequences of mixed syllables used to communicate.
Social/Play-Plays simple ball game. Imitates favorite games. Shows interest in picture books and turns pages. Is affectionate toward familiar people.

Fifteen months
Fine Motor-Places pegs and round puzzle pieces randomly. Dumps pellet from bottle on request. Stacks 2-3 cubes. Scribbles spontaneously when given crayon.
Gross Motor-Rarely falls when walking. Runs stiff-legged. Climbs on and off of chairs. Gets to standing position unaided.
Language-Uses vocabulary of 2-5 words. Points to common objects on request. Imitates easy words. Shakes head appropriately for yes and no.
Social/Play-Pulls person to show things. Uses spoon, spills good amount. Helps pull off clothes. Exhibits early tantrums.

Eighteen months
Fine Motor-Stacks 3-4 cubes. Imitates drawing straight line. Finishes small pegboard. Uses trial and error to place puzzle pieces.
Gross Motor-Walks upstairs and downstairs holding on. Kicks ball forward.
Language-Combines 2 ideas (car go, get down) (21 months) Uses jargon; 6-20 recognizable words. Points to pictures in book. Points to 4-8 body parts on request.
Social/Play-Imitates household tasks like sweeping, dusting. etc.. Takes off socks, shoes. Throws ball overhand.

Twenty-four months
Fine Motor-Stacks 6-8 cubes. Opens door. Imitates construction of simple block train. Uses visual matching of a few shapes to place puzzle pieces.

Gross Motor-Jumps both feet of floor. Walks up and down stairs alone. Runs well. Catches large ball. Language-Uses I, you, no, mine. Uses short sentences: 3-4 words. Has 50 or more words in vocabulary. Follows 2-step directions with early prepositions.
Social/Play-Feeds self, spills little. Pulls on simple garment. Parallel play. May demonstrate readiness for toilet training. Exhibits early imaginative play, exhibits limit testing, negativity.

Early object use and problem solving skills

During the ages of 6-9 months, a child explores objects in his environment and experiments with actions, which he can replicate in basic forms. For instance, he may continue to squeeze a squeaky toy to hear the noise. The child is able to find objects that are hidden as he watches. From 18-21 months, he begins to think about his actions rather than simply using trial and error to cause something to happen. The child can operate switches and understand simple cause and effect. For instance, he knows that manipulating a switch causes a toy to pop up, and can repeat this action. In this stage, the child is also able to use shapes appropriately. At 4-5 years, he has greater spatial awareness and can plan ahead, creating images in his head of basic consequences before acting.

Self-feeding skills and oral motor development

At birth, rooting, cough and gag reflexes are present. An infant can bring his hand to his mouth and can recognize a bottle. At 4-5 months, she attempts to hold the bottle with one or both hands and begins to munch with a simple bite and release. At 6 months, the infant can drink from a held cup or feed herself a cracker or biscuit as the tongue begins to strengthen. At 9 months, she can manipulate finger foods. At 12 months, the child can hold a cup and a spoon, though with some spillage. The jaw is strong enough for harder foods. At 24 months, the jaw is strong enough for most meats and vegetables, and feeding with utensils becomes more efficient. By 36 months, she can stab food with a fork and can feed herself and drink with less spillage.

Dressing, toileting, and home tasks

At 2 years old, a child is able to remove unfastened garments and can assist to pull down her pants. She can undo larger buttons. The child can tell her parent that she has restroom needs, but may need reminders to follow through with these consistently. Occasional accidents are common. In the home, she copies Mom's housekeeping activities, and helps to put her toys away when cued to initiate this.

At 5 years old, a child can dress in all basic garments without supervision, and can tie and untie her shoes. She will still need assistance with fastens that are behind her back. The child can toilet independently, including flushing and performing hygiene tasks. She will put her own toys away and is able to make the bed. She can make simple snacks, and can answer as well as talk on the phone appropriately.

Reflex Development

Moro reflex - a protective response that is present at birth. When an infant's head is dropped backwards, or if they are startled, they will extend and abduct their arms and spread their fingers.

Landau reflex - facilitates extension when the infant is prone and is present at 3-4 months. It causes extension of the head, limbs and back when the infant is held suspended and supported in a prone position.

Asymmetric Tonic Neck reflex - promotes eye-to-hand and is present at birth. It causes simultaneous extension of the arms and legs to the face and arm/leg flexion on the opposite side.

Backward Parachute reflex - promotes fall protection and is present at 9-10 months. It causes extension of one of the arms when the infant is suddenly tipped backwards.

Reflex	Appear	Disappear	Stimulus & Response
Crossed Extension	Birth	1-2 months	Noxious stimulus to the sole of one foot (stabilized.) Other leg flexes and then extends.
Flexor Withdrawal	Birth	1-2 months	Noxious stimulus to the sole; hip & knee flex; ankle dorsiflexes
Traction	Birth	2-5 months	Pull to sit grasping forearms; shoulders, elbows, wrist and fingers flex
Tonic Labyrinthian	Birth	4-6 months	Increased flexor tone when neck is extended; increased extensor tone with flexed neck.
ATNR	Birth	4-6 months	With rotation of the neck; increased extensor tone on face side; increased flexor tone on occiput side
STNR	4-6 months	8-12 months	Flexed neck-increased flexor tone of UE; increased extensor tone of LE; Extended neck; increased extensor tone of UE; Increased flexor tone of LE
Galant	Birth	2 months	Pressure on lateral spine from 12th rib to iliac crest; incurving of trunk toward side of stimulation
Moro	Birth	5-6 months	Head drops with relation to trunk; extension and abduction of arms followed by flexion and adduction
Startle	Birth	5-6 months	Same as Moro except loud noise is the stimulus
Optical Righting Reaction(RR)	Birth-2 months	Persists	Tilt upright infant and infant will right to vertical
Body on Head RR	Birth-2 months	5 years	Infant's head rights to

			vertical when placed in prone
Labyrinthine RR on head	Birth	Persists	Blindfold infant-tilt in all directions and infant's head will return to vertical
Rooting	Birth	3 months	Touch cheek to mouth; head and tongue turn toward stimulus
Suck / Swallow	Birth	2-5 months	Sucking coordinated with swallowing-stimulus is to the lips
Plantar Grasp	Birth	9 months	Press thumb into infant's foot; toes flex and adduct
Palmar Grasp	Birth	4-6 months	Press thumb into infants palm; fingers flex and adduct
Primary Standing	Birth	2 months	Stand on flat surface; extensionof knees and hips (not fully) weight bearing on legs
Stepping	Birth	2 months	Same as standing but tilt forward-heel toe stepping movements with ankle dorsiflexion, toe extension
Placing of Arms & Legs	Birth	2 months	Ankle dorsiflexor stimulation – infant lifts foot and puts it on the table; Stimulation to the back of the wrist, places hand on table
Positive Supporting Reaction-arms	3 months	4-6 months	In prone, infant bears weight on forearms (3 months) or hands with elbows and wrist extended (6 months)
Positive Supporting Reaction-legs	6-9 months	Persists	Lower child vertically so feet contact surface; child bears weight bilaterally; hips and knees extend-full wt. bearing
Protective Extension legs and arms (Parachute reaction)	4months	Persists	Thrust child toward a surface-extended arms or extended legs make contact-also can be called a positive supporting reaction
Protective Extension-fwd	6-9 months	Persists	In sitting, push infant forward-arms will go forward and plant for

- 55 -

			support.
Protective Extension-sideways	7-8 months	Persists	Push infant sideways and he will catch himself with the arm opposite the side of the push
Protective extension-backwards	9-10 months	Persists	Displace child backward and child's arms extend backwards to catch
Landau	2-4 months	1-2 years	Suspend child prone and spine will extend; scapulae adduct and arms extend and adduct
Equilibrium reactions (ER) Prone	5-6 months	Mature at 4 years	Tilt child right or left-trunk shows concavity of spine to the up side with up side limbs straightening and abduction
ER in Supine	7-8 months	Mature at 4 years	Same only supine
ER in Sitting	7-8 months	Mature at 4 years	Same-limbs on down side may go into protective extension-posterior tilting –spine is concave posteriorly, anterior tilit-spine is concave anteriorly-arms straight and abduct
Protective Staggering	15-18 months	Persists	Displace child's COG-steps in the direction being push

Grip Development

Palmar grasp - develops at five months. With this type of grip, the infant uses her fingers to push an item into her palm. The thumb is pulled in to touch the item, and the wrist may be flexed.

Radial-digital grasp - develops at 8-9 months. In this grasp, the object is held more precisely between the fingertips and the thumb, which is in opposition. The wrist is held in extension.

Inferior pincer grasp - develops at 9 months and marks the initial stage of opposition. An object is held between the distal thumb and the side of the index finger.

Fine pincer grasp - present at 12 months, when opposition has developed. The object is held between the thumb and index fingertips, or between the nails of these two digits.

Static tripod posture - a preschool writing grip that develops at 3 ½ to 4 years of age. The writing utensil is held firmly with the thumb, index and middle fingers. The hand moves to produce writing rather than the fingers.

Specific Pediatric Conditions

Wilm's tumor: kidney tumor found in children. Cause: unknown/possible genetic link. Tumor will spread to other regions. Sometimes children will be born with aniridia. Do not exert pressure over the abdomen.

Symptoms:	Tests:	Treatment:
Fever	BUN	Surgery
Vomiting	Creatinine	Chemotherapy
Fatigue	Analysis of the urine	Radiation
Irregular urine coloration	X-ray	
Abdominal pain	CT Scan	
Constipation	Family history of cancer	
Abdominal mass	CBC	
Increased BP		

Neuroblastoma: tumor in children that starts from nervous tissue. Capable of spreading rapidly. Cause unknown.

Symptoms:	Tests:
Abdominal mass	Bone scan
Skin color changes	CBC
Fatigue	MIBG scan
Tachycardia	Catecholamines tests
Motor paralysis	X-ray
Anxiety	CT scan
Diarrhea	MRI
Random eye movements	
Bone and joint pain	
Labored breathing	

Treatment:	Monitor the patient for:
Radiation	Kidney failure
Chemotherapy	Metastasis
Surgery	Various Organ system failures
	Liver failure

Cerebral palsy: Cerebrum injury causing multiple nerve function deficits. Cerebral palsy (CP) is different from other developmental disabilities due to its distinct motor components. The child with CP can have tonal abnormalities in one or more limbs, most of which involve spasticity, or hypertonia. This is characterized by exaggerated stretch reflexes, clonus, and persistent primitive reflexes and can result in decreased range of motion as well as slower fine and gross motor movements. Involuntary movements may be present, in addition to poor balance and stability. The child may be hypo- or hypersensitive to input due to lesions in the brain, which may contribute to social and/or emotional difficulties. He may also exhibit abnormal posturing such as "tailbone sitting" and habitual patterns of flexion and extension due to an inability to balance in a neutral posture. He may have difficulties with lip and tongue control, which can lead to language deficits as well as difficulty with swallowing. There is a risk of aspiration and malnutrition, and visual impairments are common.

Types:	Symptoms:
Spastic CP 50%	Poor respiration status
Dyskinetic CP 20%	Mental retardation
Mixed CP	Spasticity
Ataxic CP	Speech and language deficits
	Delayed motor and sensory development
	Seizures

Tests:	Treatment:

Sensory and Motor Skill testing
Check for spasticity
CT scan/MRI
EEG

PT/OT/ST
Surgery
Seizure medications
Spasticity reducing medicationJoint contractions

Croup: trouble breathing in infants and children that can be caused by bacteria, viruses, allergies or foreign objects. Primarily, caused by viruses.

Symptoms:
Labored breathing
Symptoms increased at night.
Noisy cough
Stridor

Tests:
X-rays
Breaths sounds check

Treatment:
Acetaminophen
Steroid medications
Intubation
Nebulizers

Monitor the patient for:
Respiratory arrest
Atelectasis
Dehydration
Epiglottitis

Kawasaki disease: a disease that affects young children primarily. Unknown origin probable autoimmune disease. Attacks the heart, blood vessels, and lymph nodes.

Symptoms:
Fever
Joint pain
Swollen lymph nodes
Peripheral edema
Rashes
Papillae on the tongue
Chapped/Red lips

Tests:
CBC
Presence of pyuria
Chest X-ray
ECGH
ESR
Urine Analysis

Treatment:
Gamma globulin
Salicylate treatment

Monitor the patient for:
Coronary aneurysm
MI
Vasculitis

Pyloric stenosis: a narrowing of the opening between the intestine and stomach. Most common in infants. May have genetic factors

Symptoms:
Diarrhea
Abdominal pain
Belching
Vomiting
Weight loss

Tests:
Abdomen distended
Barium X-ray
US
Electrolyte imbalance

Treatment:
Surgery
IV fluids

Vaccinations
Attenuated – Varicella, MMR
Inactivated – Influenza
Toxoid – Tetanus/Diptheria

- 58 -

Biosynthetic – Hib conjugate vaccine

Tetralogy of Fallot- 4 heart defects that are congenital. Poorly oxygenated blood is pumped to the body's tissues.

4 factors:	*Symptoms:*	*Tests:*
Right ventricular hypertrophy	Poor weight gain	Chest X-ray
Ventricular septal defect	Cyanosis	EKG
Aorta from both ventricles	Death	Echocardiogram
Stenosis of the pulmonic outflow tract	Limited infant feeding	Heart Catheterization
	Clubbing	CBC
	SOB	Heart Murmur

Treatment:	*Monitor the patient for:*
Surgery	Seizures
Small meals	Poor overall development
Limit child's anxiety	Cyanois

Atrial septal defect- congenital opening between the atria.

Symptoms:	*Tests:*
Dyspnea	Catheterization
Reoccurring infections (respiratory)	Echocardiography
SOB	ECG
Palpitations	MRI
	Irregular heart rhythm/sounds

Treatment:	*Monitor the patient for:*
Surgery	Heart failure
Antibiotics	A fib.
	Pulmonary Htn.
	Endocarditis

Ventricular septal defect- opening between the ventricles of the heart.

Symptoms:	*Tests:*	*Monitor the patient for:*
Poor weight gain	Ausculatation	Endocarditis
Labored breathing	Echocardiogram	Pulmonary Htn.
Profuse sweating	ECG	Aortic insufficiency
SOB	Chest X-ray	Limited growth and development
Poor color	Treatment:	Arrhythmias
Irregular heart beat	Digoxin	CHF
Respiratory infections reoccurring	Surgery	
	Digitalis	

Patent ductus arteriosus: open blood vessel (ductus ateriosus) that does not close after birth.

Symptoms:	*Tests:*
SOB	ECG
Limited feeding	Echocardiogram
	Heart murmur
	Chest X-ray

Treatment:	*Monitor the patient for:*

Surgery
Indomethacin
Decrease fluid volumes

Surgical complications
Endocarditis
Heart failure

Aortic coarctation: aorta becomes narrow at some point due to a birth defect

Symptoms:
Headache
Hypertension with activity
Nose bleeding
Fainting
SOB

Tests:
Check BP
Doppler US
Chest CT
MRI
ECG
Chest X-ray
Cardiac catheterization

Treatment:
Surgery

Monitor the patient for:
Stroke
Heart failure
Aortic aneurysm
Htn
CAD
Endocarditis
Aortic dissection

Neural tube deficit in infants

At the 3-5 month stage, healthy infants use their visual sense to explore their environments. If the infant is unable to extend the torso and lift the head, she should be placed in a carry seat with the head supported. In the 6-9 month stage, healthy infants are able to sit unsupported while they explore items in the immediate environment with their hands. A child with severe spina bifida may require a sitting jacket or a chair to maintain trunk support while allowing her to play.

At 7-12 months, healthy infants are able to scoot or crawl in order to explore the environment. An infant with postural deficits can benefit from a caster cart that provides support while allowing free movement at the floor level. At 12 months, healthy children begin to stand and walk and can explore items at eye-level. A standing brace can provide the child with a neral tube defect adequate support in this position.

Grief Process

According to Kübler-Ross, there are five stages of grief we experience after a loss, be it the loss of a friend or the losses associated with a chronic illness:

- Denial
- Anger
- Bargaining
- Depression
- Acceptance

Denial

If denial gets in the way of accepting the implications of the disease or prompt treatment, it can be a serious problem, but, for most people, denial is simply a psychological buffer against the shock of diagnosis

Level 1 : Denial of Personal Relevance
Level 2 : Denial of Urgency
Level 3 : Denial of Vulnerability
Level 4 : Denial of Feelings
Level 5 : Denial of Source of Feelings
Level 6 : Denial of Threatening Information
Level 7 : Denial of All Information

Denial is a normal response to a threatening situation, and the level of denial anyone employs will almost certainly depend on the seriousness of his or her condition.

Anger
Trying to suppress anger can lead to other problems, such as channeling resentment into resistance to treatment.

Bargaining
This period usually passes fairly quickly, if only because most people quickly realize the futility of such empty bargaining.

Depression
Everyone, healthy or not, feels a little blue at times; there'd be something wrong if they didn't. Those emotional slumps are what psychologists call 'endogenous' depression, inner storms that are usually as temporary as the weather — they might even be 'caused' by the weather, or by waking up 'on the wrong side of the bed.' The other type, 'reactive' depression, is rooted in some definable outside event, such as being diagnosed with a fatal disease.   Other emotional changes and signs of clinical depression (depression for which you should refer patients to professional help):

- Marked changes in sleeping patterns, especially having trouble sleeping at all.
- Ongoing fatigue and listlessness.
- Changes in appetite, either a loss of appetite or over-eating.
- Uncontrollable feelings of sadness, guilt, worthlessness or purposelessness.
- An inability to concentrate on anything for longer than a few moments.
- Suicidal thoughts.
- Problems with sexual function.
- Illness Intrusiveness

Acceptance
Everything — coping with an illness, learning to set new goals, getting on with life — naturally follows from acceptance.

Mental Health

Global Assessment of Functioning (GAF) Scale (DSM Axis V)

Code   Description of Functioning

91 - 100	Person has no problems OR has superior functioning in several areas OR is admired and sought after by others due to positive qualities
81 - 90	Person has few or no symptoms. Good functioning in several areas. No more than "everyday" problems or concerns.
71 - 80	Person has symptoms/problems, but they are temporary, expectable reactions to stressors. There is no more than slight impairment in any area of psychological functioning.
61 - 70	Mild symptoms in one area OR difficulty in one of the following: social, occupational, or school functioning. BUT, the person is generally functioning pretty well and has some meaningful interpersonal relationships.
51 - 60	Moderate symptoms OR moderate difficulty in one of the following: social, occupational, or school functioning.
41 - 50	Serious symptoms OR serious impairment in one of the following: social, occupational, or school functioning.
31 - 40	Some impairment in reality testing OR impairment in speech and communication OR serious impairment in several of the following: occupational or school functioning, interpersonal relationships, judgment, thinking, or mood.
21 - 30	Presence of hallucinations or delusions which influence behavior OR serious impairment in ability to communicate with others OR serious impairment in judgment OR inability to function in almost all areas.
11 - 20	There is some danger of harm to self or others OR occasional failure to maintain personal hygiene OR the person is virtually unable to communicate with others due to being incoherent or mute.
1 - 10	Persistent danger of harming self or others OR persistent inability to maintain personal hygiene OR person has made a serious attempt at suicide.

Mental Retardation

Mild MR is classified as an IQ range of 55-69. These individuals require minimal assistance to function in society due to decreased social skills and need for vocational training. Some will need intermittent support to live independently.

In moderate MR, the IQ ranges 40-54. These individuals require daily support limited to specific performance areas, i.e. housekeeping skills. They can function in a basic routine with supervisory checks, and can work under guidance.

In severe MR, the IQ ranges from 25-39. These individuals must be supervised for all aspects of the daily routine, and will need assistance with ADLS. Communication skills are usually impaired.

In profound MR, the IQ is less than 25. These individuals will need assistance with all aspects of their daily routine, and may have severe physical developmental impairments.

All individuals with MR have a risk of sensory impairments such as visual deficits, in addition to a risk for seizures.

Attention-Deficit/Hyperactivity Disorder

Occupational therapy for the child with Attention-Deficit/Hyperactivity Disorder, or ADHD, should be focused both on the home and school environments in order to help provide necessary structure. This is needed to encourage successful performance of the child as well as to facilitate community integration. The OT may teach the child strategies for self-control, as well as anger and excitement management. Sensory modulation is also important, so that the child can learn to multi-process without being overwhelmed. Social skills training may be necessary in order to facilitate the child's participation in social groups and play with peers. During treatment, it is important that the OT maintain open communication with parents and teachers for carryover of skills and coping strategies taught during therapy sessions. Teachers and parents should be encouraged to provide feedback about the child's performance in the absence of the therapist, and should demonstrate competence with enforcement of strategies taught by the OT.

Paranoid schizophrenia

Positive symptoms of paranoid schizophrenia include auditory or visual hallucinations, grandiose delusions and incoherent speech and thought process. Negative symptoms include flat affect, decreased initiation of activity, and poor eye contact. A patient with paranoid schizophrenia will have difficulty engaging in goal-directed activities, and tends to lack adequate social skills. He may have difficulties completing basic or advanced ADLs due to thought disorder and/or cognitive deficits.

OT intervention is focused on maintaining existing functional skills, as well as developing the skills needed for survival. Engaging the patient in group activities is appropriate to assist in development of social interaction skills. It is also important to establish a routine for basic and advanced ADLs. Community reintegration should be initiated with patients who are planning to be discharged from the hospital, and should focus on involvement in work, school and home management tasks.

Borderline personality disorder

A patient with borderline personality disorder typically has an unstable mood and is quick to anger. This makes behavior unpredictable, and she may drive people away due to her actions. In the clinical setting, she might have a love-hate type relationship with staff, and tend to use splitting as a way to get control over her situation.

When an OT is faced with treating a patient with borderline personality disorder, she must keep control over the treatment session and not allow herself to get upset over the patient's actions or words. Establishing rules or guidelines with the team and the patient is a good place to start. The therapist must clearly spell out what she expects from the patient, and must be firm with the behavior program that is established. A schedule for therapy sessions will be useful. Once the patient is participating, positive reinforcement through praise and rewards can help keep the patient on track.

Mental health terms

Learned helplessness is the sense of a loss of control over events in one's life. A patient who is experiencing learned helplessness feels that no matter what she does, her situation will not change. In treatment, this often reflects a loss of insight.

Self-prediction is the anticipation of one's performance on a task prior to its completion. This includes not only the ability to complete the task, but also the components of task such as the estimated time that will required to complete it. A patient with a deficit in this area may underestimate or overestimate her abilities, or the level of assistance she may require.

Self-evaluation is the ability to rate one's own performance of a particular task. A patient can review her own actions, and consider potential changes to ease the future performance of this task.

Anorexia nervosa

According to the American Psychological Association, there are four criteria for a diagnosis of anorexia nervosa:
1. The patient's weight is less than 85% of the norm for age, height and build.
2. The patient is obsessive about her weight, or becoming "fat". She considers weight loss to be an achievement tied to self-esteem.
3. The patient's body image is distorted, and she may still consider herself overweight even when she is clearly underweight.
4. The patient has missed three or more menstrual cycles.

OT goals for patients with anorexia nervosa are to restore weight as closely as possible to norms, to restore the menstrual cycle, to establish normal eating patterns, and to address the underlying psychological factors of the disorder. Some useful interventions are assertiveness training, appropriate use of exercise (as opposed to overuse), expressive activities such as art or dance, involvement in leisure activity and nutritional education.

Bulimia nervosa

According to the American Psychological Association, the four diagnostic criteria for bulimia nervosa are:
1. Periods of binging, with a lack of control over how much and what kinds of food are eaten.
2. Excessive exercise, or use of vomiting, diuretics or laxatives to compensate for episodes binging.
3. Cycles of binging and purging behaviors have occurred a minimum of twice a week for a period of at least 12 weeks.
4. An unreasonable association of weight and body shape with self-esteem.

OT goals for a patient with bulimia nervosa are similar to those for anorexia nervosa, and include restoration of normal eating patterns, treatment of associated psychological disorders and challenging associated values. Cognitive behavioral treatment can be effective in developing healthy attitudes about body image and self-esteem. Expressive therapies can also be useful.

Learning disabilities

Children with learning disabilities often have deficits in motor performance, as well as poorly integrated vestibular and/or proprioceptive input. They may have a poor ability to adequately grasp a pencil, leading to irregularities in lettering. Attention may be diminished, which can lead to disorganized completion of assignments. Participation in group activities may be poor due to insecurity with physical performance. This can cause difficulty in establishing and maintaining friendships within peer groups.

The OT must identify the sensory integration deficits, and address these performance components. Performing standardized tests, in addition to interviewing family and/or teachers, can help establish areas that need remediation. The overall goals are usually to increase the child's ability to process sensory information, to teach compensatory strategies for underlying deficits, and to make or suggest environmental adaptations.

Substance abuse

Patients who have undergone treatment for substance abuse may benefit from group treatments to facilitate social skills training and to decrease feelings of social isolation, which are common in his client group. Patients may benefit from practicing assertiveness and communication skills to encourage positive social interaction experiences.

OT will also need to focus on the areas of life skills training, with particular emphasis on home management tasks. Cleanliness, money management, and IADL planning are generally impaired in this client group. These patients will benefit from budget training and meal planning, in addition to safety awareness and complex problem solving related to the home environment.

With regards to work, OT intervention should focus on high level problem solving skills as well as the physical factors of a potential job, such as fine and gross coordination. Practice of job interview skills may be appropriate.

Task attention

There are four levels of task attention:
- Sustained attention is the process of staying focused on a task for the duration of the activity. A patient with a deficit in this area might tend to leave tasks in various states of completion.
- Selective attention is the process of focusing on one task in the presence of competing stimuli. A patient with a deficit in this area might get distracted while trying to focus on an activity in a noisy room.
- Divided attention is the process of focusing on more than one task during a designated time. A patient with a deficit in this area will have trouble multitasking.
- Alternating attention is the process of redirecting attention between two tasks. A patient with a deficit in this area might have difficulty spontaneously resuming a laundry task after to answering a knock at the door.

Assessing cognition

Orientation can be simply tested by asking the patient to state his name, where he is, and what is happening. Often these questions are repeated to patients throughout the stay in any given facility, and it is possible for the answers to be memorized. A patient can also be asked to describe their schedule, or the routine tasks that are performed by hospital personnel.

Attention can be easily assessed by asking the patient to participate in tasks such as crossing out letters, or in basic ADLs. The OT should watch for signs of distractibility during performance. Memory can be assessed by asking the patient to recall the name of the facility, their nurse or therapist. The OT can also present the patient with several objects during evaluation, and later ask the patient to recall as many as possible.

Sensory integration

Sensory integration is often performed with children who have deficits in age-appropriate movements and sensation. It is often performed with specialized play equipment, which encourages the child to complete certain remedial movements in order to perform the activity. For instance, a child may be taken through an obstacle course of ramps and pulleys in order to challenge postural responses. Multi-sensory experiences are encouraged in this approach, such as visual integration of the activity. SI can also address deficits in sensation including tactile defensiveness.

When treating a child using SI, the therapist should take care to use equipment that is age-appropriate and durable. Most SI equipment is for use during guided play, and can appear exciting to young patients. Care should be taken to provide continual supervision in the SI environment to ensure that equipment is used properly and safely.

Hypersensitivity

A patient with a hypersensitive limb is at risk for disability due to decreased use of the affected extremity during functional tasks that cause pain. In addition to desensitization training, the patient may benefit from compensatory training. A patient can be taught to handle items so that areas of concentrated pressure are avoided. Repetitive motions should be avoided to decrease friction, and protective garments such as gloves or long sleeves may be useful. Education regarding careful handling of sharp objects in addition to sources of heat or cold can aid the patient in motor planning to decrease the noxious affects of such items. Finally, the patient should be taught to rely on other senses such as vision and hearing to make themselves aware of potential hazards.

Stages of Dementia Analysis (Reisburg)

CONCENTRATION: (1) no objective or subjective evidence of deficit; (2) subjective decrement; (3) minor objective signs –7s; (4) definite deficit for person of their background; (5) marked deficit - 2sl (6) forgets the concentration task; (7) marked difficulty counting 1-10.

RECENT MEMORY: (1) no objective or subjective evidence; (2) subjective impairment only; (3) deficit in recall of specific events upon detailed questioning; (4) cannot recall major events of previous weekend or week; (5) occasional knowledge of some events. (6) Little or no idea of current address, weather, etc. (7) no knowledge of any recent events.

PAST MEMORY: (1) No objective or subjective evidence; (2) subjective impairment only; (3) some gaps in past memory upon detailed questioning; (4) clear-cut deficit. Spouse recalls more of the pts past. Cannot recall childhood friends and/or teachers. Confuses chronology. (5) major past events sometimes not recalled; (6) some residual memory of past (e.g. birthplace or occupation); (7) no memory of past.

ORIENTATION: (1) no deficit; (2) subjective impairment; (3) any mistakes in time >2 hrs, day of week >1 day, date > 3 days; (4) mistakes in month >10 days or year >1 month; (5) unsure of month and/or year and/or season; unsure of locale; (6) no idea of date. Identifies spouse but may not recall name. Knows own name. (7) can not identify spouse. May be unsure of personal identity.

FUNCTIONING & SELF-CARE: (1) none; (2) forgets location of objects; (3) decreased job function. Difficulty traveling to new place. (4) Decreased ability to perform complex tasks; (5) Requires assistance in choosing proper clothing; (6) requires assistance in feeding and/or toileting and/or bathing and/or ambulating; (7) requires constant assistance in all ADLs.

TOTAL SCORE

Stage on (GDS) , Global Deterioration Scale

Dementia

A condition characterized by the loss of basic cognitive and physical functions such as reasoning, short-term memory, posture and ambulation, logic, sequencing and performance of self-care tasks. The causes of dementia are variable, but are usually related to permanent changes in the central nervous system. It is generally progressive.

Delirium

A condition characterized by a change in cognition, decreased perceptual abilities or the loss of the ability to focus. It generally has a more acute onset than dementia, though can be long-lasting depending on the cause. Delirium can be a sign of dementia or a psychiatric disorder, but it can also be triggered by drug reactions, severe fatigue, or an anxiety attack. Delirium is usually resolvable, thought some deficits may remain due to the underlying cause.

Alternatives to restraints

Many patients who are confused tend to wander, and may be unable to locate familiar areas, which can have dangerous consequences. For the elderly in skilled facilities, rooms should be clearly marked, and repetition should be used to establish locations of safe areas. A wander guard that alarms when a patient reaches a certain zone can ensure that these patients do not leave the unit unnoticed. This is preferable to a restraint. Supervision is often necessary, and structured programs or environments can be useful in preventing patients from becoming agitated or getting lost. Some facilities provide safe wandering areas for patients who like to walk. For the patient who needs assistance with ADLs, regular checks for toileting needs can help prevent many falls and will decrease the need for a restraint.

Paranoid schizophrenia

Positive symptoms of paranoid schizophrenia include auditory or visual hallucinations, grandiose delusions and incoherent speech and thought process. Negative symptoms include flat affect, decreased initiation of activity, and poor eye contact. A patient with paranoid schizophrenia will have difficulty engaging in goal-directed activities, and tends to lack adequate social skills. He may have difficulties completing basic or advanced ADLs due to thought disorder and/or cognitive deficits. OT intervention is focused on maintaining existing functional skills, as well as developing the skills needed for survival. Engaging the patient in group activities is appropriate to assist in development of social interaction skills. It is also important to establish a routine for basic and advanced ADLs. Community reintegration should be initiated with patients who are planning to be discharged from the hospital, and should focus on involvement in work, school and home management tasks.

Extrapyramidal symptoms (EPS)

EPS is common side effect of some of the more traditional anti-psychotic medications, and they often appear in patients who are taking such drugs to control the symptoms of schizophrenia. These side effects include tardive diskinesia, in which patients experience involuntary movements of the mouth, such as rolling the tongue around or repeatedly licking the lips. Facial tics may be present. A patient may also demonstrate akathisia, which is an involuntary need to be moving constantly. The patient may appear fidgety, or unable to sit quietly. Pacing is common with EPS. Another sign of EPS is acute dystonia, in which muscle groups contract involuntarily. These contractions can cause pain. EPS can appear in various degrees of severity at any time during antipsychotic drug use, and may resolve if the drugs are discontinued.

Grandiose delusions
A patient may be having grandiose delusions if he has an inflated sense of importance beyond his reality. He may think he is a famous rock star, or that he is a close, personal friend of someone who holds high power. Sometimes the patient may think he is supremely knowledgeable, or even omnipotent.

Magical thinking
Magical thinking involves linking extraordinary traits or abilities with common objects or actions. In other words, a patient may believe that a particular hat can keep people from reading his thoughts, or that an object such as a necklace offers him protection.

Paranoid ideation
Paranoid ideation is the persistent belief that one is being persecuted, or is a target for suspicious activities. A patient who is paranoid may think that he is being chased or followed, or may claim that his thoughts or actions are being monitored. Most paranoid ideas in patients who have psychosis are unrealistic.

Developmental Theories

Characteristics of Play
12-24 months
Children participate in symbolic play. This is characterized by "make believe" play and is primarily focused on basic self-care tasks such as eating or washing. Children may mimic familiar tasks in an unrealistic way, such as attempting to feed a stuffed animal, or using a ball as a car. Symbolic play continues to develop through age 4 as children begin to involve their peers in this form of play.

4-7 years
Children participate in creative play, which is characterized by peer groups and social interaction. In creative play there is focus on motor skill development and laying foundations for school related activities.

7-10 years
Children begin to participate in game play with focus on following rules and being in competition with peers. Social interaction in this stage fosters friendship as peer groups gain importance.

Erik Erikson's 8 Stages of Psychosocial Development

Erik Erikson defined eight stages of development, each with a crisis that must be resolved in order to master the stage and move to the next level. Each level provides a necessary personal quality to the individual. Erikson's stages are as follows: basic trust vs. mistrust, for meeting basic survival needs (infancy); autonomy vs. doubt, in which the child gains bodily control (2-4 years); initiative vs. guilt, for social skills development (preschool); industry vs. inferiority, in which competency is achieved (elementary), self-identity vs. role diffusion, for societal integration (teenage); intimacy vs. isolation, in which partnerships are established (early adulthood); generativity vs. self-absorption, for professional roles (adulthood); and integrity vs. despair, for reflection on life (elderly).

Stage	Ages	Basic Conflict	Important Event	Summary
1. Oral-Sensory	Birth to 12 to 18 months	Trust vs. Mistrust	Feeding	The infant must form a first loving, trustingrelationship with the caregiver, or develop a sense of mistrust.
2.Muscular-Anal	18 months to 3years	Autonomy vs. Shame/Doubt	Toilet training	Thechild's energies are directed toward the development of physical skills,including walking, grasping, and rectal sphincter control. The child learnscontrol but may develop shame and doubt if not handled well.
3. Locomotor	3 to 6 years	Initiativevs. Guilt	Independence	The child continues to become more assertive and to take moreinitiative, but may be too forceful, leading to guilt feelings.
4. Latency	6 to 12 years	Industryvs. Inferiority	School	Thechild must deal with demands to learn new skills or risk a sense of inferiority,failure and incompetence.
6. Young Adulthood	19 to 40 years	Intimacyvs. Isolation	Love relationships	The young adult must develop intimate relationships or sufferfeelings of isolation.

Piaget's Cognitive Development Review

Jean Piaget felt that maturation was dependent upon physical growth in the endocrine and nervous systems, with experiences and social interactions. Piaget organizes development into the following stages:

Sensorimotor period - 0-2 years
- development of action schemes

Preoperational period - 2-7 years
- child begins to deal with mental representations
- egocentric view – doesn't realize that others view the social and physical environment differently from them
- no understanding of differing perspectives
- reliance on centration - tendency to focus on a single detail of a question or problem and subsequently to be unable to shift to another detail or dimension

Period of concrete operations 7-11 years
- increased sensitivity to contradictions inherent in his/her own thoughts
- beginnings of ability to make judgments on the basis of his/her conception of the meaning behind various perceptions rather than on the basis of perception alone
- able to understand relationships among specific events in the environment
- not able to produce formal, abstract hypotheses

- 69 -

- cannot image possible events that are not also real events, thus cannot solve problems that involve formal abstractions
- bound up with the world as it is

Period of formal operations 11+
- begin to display the ability to engage in formal reasoning on an abstract level
- can imagine hypothetical as well as real events
- begin to consider all possible explanations to a problem and only then do they try to discover, systematically, which of the explanations really applies
- begin to understand that what occurs in reality is just one among many possible alternatives

Maslow's Hierarchy of Needs

In the levels of the five basic needs, the person does not feel the second need until the demands of the first have been satisfied, nor the third until the second has been satisfied, and so on. Maslow's basic needs are as follows:

Physiological Needs
These are biological needs. They consist of needs for oxygen, food, water, and a relatively constant body temperature. They are the strongest needs because if a person were deprived of all needs, the physiological ones would come first in the person's search for satisfaction.

Safety Needs
When all physiological needs are satisfied and are no longer controlling thoughts and behaviors, the needs for security can become active. Adults have little awareness of their security needs except in times of emergency or periods of disorganization in the social structure (such as widespread rioting). Children often display the signs of insecurity and the need to be safe.

Needs of Love, Affection and Belongingness
When the needs for safety and for physiological well-being are satisfied, the next class of needs for love, affection and belongingness can emerge. Maslow states that people seek to overcome feelings of loneliness and alienation. This involves both giving and receiving love, affection and the sense of belonging.

Needs for Esteem
When the first three classes of needs are satisfied, the needs for esteem can become dominant. These involve needs for both self-esteem and for the esteem a person gets from others. Humans have a need for a stable, firmly based, high level of self-respect, and respect from others. When these needs are satisfied, the person feels self-confident and valuable as a person in the world. When these needs are frustrated, the person feels inferior, weak, helpless and worthless.

Needs for Self-Actualization
When all of the foregoing needs are satisfied, then and only then are the needs for self-actualization activated. Maslow describes self-actualization as a person's need to be and do that which the person was "born to do." "A musician must make music, an artist must paint, and a poet must write." These needs make themselves felt in signs of restlessness.

Adaptive skills

Ann Mosey defined six major adaptive skills that are important to occupational performance.

1. Sensory integration of input for use in function: this involves the tactile system, proprioception, body scheme awareness, motor planning of fine and gross movements, and vestibular reactions.
2. Cognitive skills: these involve perception, deliberate actions and trial and error, representation and organization of sensory information, problem solving and environmental exploration.
3. Dyadic interaction skill: this is the ability to participate in relationships, including family, friends, playmates, peers, and authority figures.
4. Group interaction skills: these refer to the ability to participate in various types of groups including parallel, cooperative, egocentric, project-related and mature groups.
5. Self-identity skill: this involves perception of the self as a valued person who is an independent contributing member of society. It includes the understanding that death is a necessary part of life.
6. Sexual identity skill: this involves feeling comfortable with one's changing sexual nature, taking into account mutual satisfaction and age-related physiology.

GI Review

GI Conditions

Zollinger-Ellison syndrome: Tumors of the pancreas that cause upper GI inflammation. The tumors secrete gastrin causing high levels of stomach acid.

Symptoms:	*Tests:*	*Treatment:*
Diarrhea	Abdominal CT	Ranitidine
Vomiting	+ Calcium Infusion Test	Cimetidine
Abdominal pain	+ Secretin Stimulation Test	Lansoprazole
	Elevated gastrin levels	Omeprazole
	Tumors in the pancreas	Surgery

Wilson's disease: High levels of copper in various tissues throughout the body. (Genetically linked-Autosomal recessive).

Key organs affected are:	*Symptoms:*	*Tests:*
Eyes	Gait disturbances	Various lab tests:
Brain	Jaundice	Bilirubin/PT/ SGOT increased
Liver	Tremors	Albumin/Uric acid production
Kidneys	Abdominal pain/distention	decreased
	Dementia	MRI
	Speech problems	Genetic testing
	Muscle weakness	Copper levels
	Spenomegaly	Kayser-Fleisher Rings in the eye
	Confusion	
	Dementia	

Treatment:	*Monitor the patient for:*
Pyridoxine	Cirrhosis
Low copper diet	Muscle weakness
Corticosteroids	Joint pain/stiffness
Penicillamine	Anemia
	Fever
	Hepatitis

Pancreatitis: Inflammation of the pancreas

Symptoms:	Tests:
Fever	X-ray
Vomiting	CT scan
Nausea	Various Lab tests
Chills	
Anxiety	
Jaundice	
Sweating	

Pancreatic Cancer: cancer of the pancreas. Higher rates in men.

Symptoms:	Tests:	Treatment:
Nausea	CT scan	Surgery
Jaundice	Biopsy	Chemotherapy
Depression	Abdominal US	Radiation
Back pain	Liver function test	Whipple procedure
Indigestion		
Abdominal pain		
Weight loss		

Hepatitis A: Viral infection that causes liver swelling.

Symptoms:	Tests:	Treatment:
Fatigue	Increased liver enzymes	Rest
Nausea	Presence of IgG and IgM	Proper diet low in fatty foods
Fever	antibodies	
Itching	Enlarged liver	
Vomiting		

Hepatitis B: Sexually transmitted disease, also transmitted with body fluids and some individual may be symptom free but still be carriers.

Symptoms:	Tests:	Treatment:
Jaundice	Decreased albumin levels	Monitor for changes in the liver.
Dark Urine	+ antibodies and antigen	Recombinant alpha interferon in some cases.
Malaise	Increased levels of transaminase	Transplant necessary if liver failure occurs.
Joint pain		
Fever		
Fatigue		

Hepatitis C

Symptoms:	Tests:	Treatment:
Fatigue	ELISA assay	Interferon alpha
Vomiting	Increased levels of liver enzymes	Ribavirin
Urine color changes (dark)	No Hep. A or B antibodies	
Jaundice		
Abdominal pain		

Gastritis: can be caused by various sources (bacteria, viruses, bile reflux or autoimmune diseases). Inflammation of the stomach lining.

Symptoms:	Tests:

Loss of appetite
Hiccups
Nausea
Vomiting blood
Abdominal pain

EGC
X-Ray
CT scan

Ulcers
Peptic Ulcers-ulcer in the duodenum or stomach
Gastric Ulcers- ulcer in the stomach
Duodenum Ulcer-ulcer in the duodenum

Bacteria: Helicobacter pylori- often associated with ulcer formation.

Symptoms:	Tests:	Treatment:
Weight loss	EGD	Bismuth
Chest pain	Stool guaiac	Famotidine
Heartburn	GI X-rays	Sucralfate
Vomiting		Cimetidine
Indigestion		Omeprazole
Fatigue		Antibiotics

Diverticulitis – abnormal pouch formation that becomes inflamed in the intestinal wall.

Symptoms:	Tests:
Fever	Barium enema
Diarrhea	WBC count
Nausea	Colonoscopy
Vomiting	CT Scan
Constipation	

Intestinal obstruction: Can a paralytic ileus/false obstruction (children) or a mechanical obstruction:

Types of mechanical obstruction:	Symptoms:	Tests:
Tumors	Constipation	Barium enema
Volvulus	Vomiting	CT scan
Impacted condition	Diarrhea	Upper/Lower GI series
Hernia	Breath	Poor bowel sounds
	Abdominal swelling	
	Abdominal pain	

Carcinoid Syndrome: symptoms caused by cardinoid tumors. Linked to increased secretion of Serotonin.

Symptoms:	Tests:
Flush appearance	5-HIAA test
Wheezing	Increased levels of Chromogranin A and Serotonin
Diarrhea	CT scan
Onset of niacin deficiency	MRI
Abdominal pain	
Decreased BP	

Treatment:	Monitor the patient for:
Surgery	Low BP

- 73 -

Sandostatin   Right Sided Heart Failure
Chemotherapy
Multivitamins
Octreotide
Interferon

Hiatal Hernia: Stomach sticks into the chest through the diaphragm. Can cause reflux symptoms.

Symptoms:	*Tests:*	*Treatment:*
Chest pain	EGD	Weight loss
Heartburn	Barium Swallow X-ray.	Surgical repair
Poor swallow		Medications for reflux

(GERD) -Gastroesophageal reflux disease

Symptoms:

Nausea	Belching	*Tests:*
Vomiting	Chest pain	Barium swallow
Frequent coughing	Anatacid relief	Bernstein test
Hoarseness	Sore Throat	Stool guaiac
		Endoscopy

Treatment:	*Monitor the patient for:*
Weight loss	Chronic pulmonary disease
Antacids	Barrett's esophagus
Proton pump inhibitors	Esophagus inflammation
Limit fat and caffeine	Bronchospasms
Histamine H2 blockers	

Ulcerative colitis: chronic inflammation of the rectum and large intestine.

Symptoms:	*Tests:*
Weight loss	Barium edema
Jaundice	ESR
Diarrhea	CRP
Abdominal pain	Colonoscopy
Fever	
Joint pain	
GI bleeding	

Treatment:	*Monitor the patient for:*
Corticosteroids	Ankylosing spondylitis
Mesalamine	Liver disease
Surgery	Carcinoma
Ostomy	Pyoderma gangrenosum
Azathioprine	Hemorrhage
	Perforated colon

Neurogenic bowel: the inability to empty the bowels without assistance. In patients with a complete spinal cord injury (SCI), a bowel program must be established in order for this function to occur. A bowel program can be completed in bed, however it is best completed on a bedside commode to encourage complete evacuation assisted by gravity. Some patients require the use of a suppository, and/or digital stimulation of the anal sphincter. A drop-arm commode is also appropriate for access

- 74 -

via slide board, and a cushioned surface such as padding is recommended for skin integrity. Failure to complete bowel or bladder evacuation can lead to autonomic dysreflexia, in addition to other medical complications such as bowel obstruction or sepsis.

Liver Function

Endocrine function
1. In response to growth hormone, the liver secretes insulin-like growth factor (IGF-I), which promotes growth by stimulating cell division in various tissues, including bone.
2. Contributes to the activation of vitamin D
3. Forms triiodothyronine T3 from thyroxine T4
4. Secretes angiotensinogen, which is acted upon by renin to form angiotensin I
5. Metabolizes hormones
A. Clotting functions
1. Produces many of the plasma clotting factors, including prothrombin and fibrinogen
2. Produces bile salts, which are essential for the gastrointestinal absorption of vitamin K, which is, in turn, needed for production of the clotting factors.

Plasma proteins
1. Synthesizes and secretes plasma albumin, acute phase proteins, binding proteins for steroid hormones and trace elements, lipoproteins, and other proteins

Exocrine functions
1. Synthesizes and secretes bile salts, which are necessary for adequate digestion and absorption of fats.
2. Secretes into the bile a bicarbonate-rich solution of inorganic ions, which helps neutralize acid in the duodenum.

Organic metabolism
1. Converts plasma glucose into glycogen and triacylglycerols during absorptive period
2. Converts plasma amino acids to fatty acids, which can be incorporated into triacylglycerols during absorptive period.
3. Synthesizes triacylglycerols and other sources during postabsorptive period and releases glucose into the blood.
4. Converts fatty acids into ketones during fasting.
5. Produces urea, the major end product of amino acid catabolism and releases it into the blood.

Cholesterol metabolism
1. Synthesizes cholesterol and releases it into the blood.
2. Secrets plasma cholesterol into the bile.
3. Converts plasma cholesterol into bile salts.

Excretory and degradative functions
1. Secretes bilirubin and other bile pigments into the bile.
2. Excretes, via the bile, many endogenous and foreign organic molecules as well as trace metals.
3. Biotransforms many endogenous and foreign organic molecules.
4. Destroys old erythrocytes.

Kidney and Urinary System

The kidneys regulate the water and ionic composition of the body, excrete waste products, excrete foreign chemicals, produce glucose during prolonged fasting, and secrete three hormones-renin, 1,25 dihydroxyvitamin D3, and erythropoietin. The first three functions are accomplished by continuous processing of the plasma. Each renal corpuscle comprises a glomerulus, and a Bowman's capsule, into which the glomerulus protrudes.

The tubule extends out from Bowman's capsule and is subdivided into many segments, which can be combined for reference purposes into the proximal tubule, loop of Henley, distal convoluted tubule, and collecting duct. Beginning at the level of the collecting ducts, multiple tubules join and empty into the renal pelvis, from which urine flows through ureters to the bladder. Each glomerulus is supplied by an afferent arteriole, and an efferent arteriole leaves the glomerulus to branch into peritubular capillaries, which supply the tubule.

The three basic renal processes are glomerular filtration, tubular reabsorption, and tubular secretion. In addition, the kidneys synthesize and/or catabolize certain substances. The excretion of a substance is equal to the amount filtered plus the amount secreted minus the amount reabsorbed.

Neurogenic bladder: the inability to void the bladder without assistance. Patients with a complete SCI require intermittent catheterization every 4-6 hours to effectively empty the bladder.
Failure to complete bowel or bladder evacuation can lead to autonomic dysreflexia, in addition to other medical complications such as bowel obstruction or sepsis.

Eye, Ear, and Mouth Review

Disorders of the Eye

Diabetic retinopathy
Blood vessels in the retina are affected. Can lead to blindness if untreated. Two primary stages (Proliferative and Nonproliferative. Retina may experience bleeding in nonproliferative stage. During the proliferative stage damage begins moving towards the center of the eye and there is an increase in bleeding. Any damage caused is non-reversible. Only further damage can be prevented.

Strabismus
Eyes are moving in different stages. The axes of the eyes are not parallel. Normally, treated with an eyepatch; however, eye drops are now used in many cases. Atropine drops are placed in the stronger eye for correction purposes. Surgery may be necessary in some cases. Suture surgery will reduce the pull of certain eye muscles.

Macular Degeneration:
Impaired central vision caused by destruction of the macula, which is the center part of the retina. Limited vision straight ahead. More common in people over 60. Can be characterized as dry or wet types. Wet type more common. Vitamin C, Zinc, and Vitamin E may help slow progression.

Esotropia:
Appearance of cross-eyed gaze or internal strabismus.

Exotropia:
External strabismus or divergent gaze.

Conjunctivitis:
Inflammation of the conjuctiva, that can be caused by viruses or bacteria. Also known as pink eye. If viral source can be highly contagious. Antibiotic eye drops and warm cloths to the eye helpful treatment. Conjunctivitis can also be caused by chemicals or allergic reactions. Re-occurring conjunctivitis can indicate a larger underlying disease process.

Glaucoma:
An increase in fluid pressure in the eye leading to possible optic nerve damage. More common in African-Americans. Minimal onset symptoms, often picked to late. Certain drugs may decrease the amount of fluid entering the eye. Two major types of glaucoma are open-angle glaucoma and \angle-closure glaucoma.

Effects of Poor Vision

Reading Ability
- Normal vision and near normal version refer to the ability to read at standard distance, or by bringing the reading material slightly closer to the face. Glasses are not needed.
- Low vision is vision that is not adequate for a person's needs without assistive devices. It is divided into three categories.
  - A patient with moderately low version would need to bring a book closer to the face, eventually causing eye discomfort. Corrective lenses will help a patient with moderately low vision.
  - A patient with severely low vision must bring a book so close to the face that only one eye will be functional to read. A strong magnifying glass may be useful in this case.
  - A patient with profoundly low vision requires the use of video magnification, or must use alternatives to reading.
- Near blindness refers to the condition in which vision is not reliable, and reading is not possible. Reading alternatives such as books on tape are necessary. With total blindness, there is no vision at all.

Self-care
- Basic self-care tasks can generally be completed with little difficulty by a patient who has low vision. Memorization of object location and limitation of items used are helpful in easing ADLs.
- Like objects should be stored together, such as an electric shaver and a toothbrush. Like-colored garments should be sorted, and stored in different parts of the closet to ease clothing selection.
- In order to ease feeding, a helper can describe the placement of items on the tray using the clock method (i.e. milk is at 1 o'clock).
- Patients should have either a large-button telephone, or a speed-dial system that they can operate in order to ensure they can to contact someone in the event of an emergency.
- Many specialized, gadget-like items that help compensate for varying degrees of visual deficits can be purchased through organizations for the blind.

Occulomotor dysfunction

A patient with occulomotor dysfunction will have deficits in eye ROM, saccades and pursuit. The patient will have trouble reading an entire page, and might see letters in a jumble or describe words "jumping off the page". An L-shaped bookmark or a typoscope bookmark can frame one sentence at a time to allow the patient to focus. The patient should be instructed to begin the sentence at the left edge of the bookmark, moving the bookmark to the right or down as appropriate.

When teaching the patient to scan, it can be helpful to place markers, such as colored tape, in important areas for the patient to seek. The patient should also practice organized scanning movements such as left to right and circular patterns to increase spatial awareness.
Eye to hand coordination should also be practiced to improve speed and accuracy of movements, which will assist function in ADL tasks and improve dexterity for fastens and gross movements. This can be achieved through remediation, or with practice of ADL tasks themselves.

Disorders of the Mouth

- Acute pharyngitis
  Often the cause of sore throats, inflammation of the pharynx.
- Acute tonsillitis
  Viral or Bacterial infection that causes inflammation of the tonsils.
- Aphthous ulcer
  Also known as a canker sore. A sensitive ulcer in the lining of the mouth. 1 in 5 people have these ulcers. Cause is unknown in many cases.
- Bottom of Form
- Acute Epiglottitis
  Inflammation of the epiglotitis that may lead to blockage of the respiratory system and death if not treated. Often caused by numerous bacteria. Intubation may be required and speed is critical in treatment. IV antibiotics will help reverse this condition in most cases. Common symptoms are high fever and sore throat.
- Oral candidiasis
  This is a yeast infection of the throat and mouth by Candida albicans.
- Oral leukoplakia
  A patch or spot in the mouth that can become cancerous.
- Parotitis
  A feature of mumps and inflammation of the parotid glands.

Disorders of the Ear

- Otitis media
  Most common caused by the bacteria (H.flu) and Streptococcus pneumoniae in about 85% of cases. 15% of cases viral related. More common in bottlefeeding babies. Can be caused by upper respiratory infections. Ear drums can rupture in severe cases. A myringotomy may be performed in severe cases to relieve pus in the middle ear.
- Barotitis
  Atmospheric pressures causing middle ear dysfunction. Any change in altitude causes problems.
- Mastoiditis

May be caused by an ear infection and is known as inflammation of the mastoid.
- Meniere's disease

    Inner ear disorder. Causes unknown. Episodic rotational vertigo, Tinnitus, Hearing loss, and Ringing in the ears are key symptoms. Dazide is the primary medication for Meniere's disease. Low salt diet and surgery are also other treatment options. Diagnosis is a rule-out diagnosis.
- Labyrinthitis

    Vertigo associated with nausea and malaise. Related to bacterial and viral infections. Inflammation of the labyrinth in the inner ear.
- Otitis externa

    Usually caused by a bacterial infection. Swimmer's ear. Infection of the skin with the outer ear canal that progress to the ear drum. Itching, Drainage and Pain are the key symptoms. Suctioning of the ear canal may be necessary. Most common ear drops (Volsol, Cipro, Cortisporin).

Obstetrics/Gynecology Review

Obstetric Tests

Amniocentesis: Removal of some fluid surrounding the fetus for analysis. Fetus location is identified by US prior to the procedure. Results may take a month.
Used to check for:
- Spina bifida
- Rh compatibility
- Immature lungs
- Down syndrome

Chorionic villus sampling: Removal of placental tissue for analysis from the uterus during early pregnancy. US helps guide the procedure. 1-2 weeks get the results. Can be performed earlier than amniocentesis.

Used to check for:	*Monitor the patient for:*
Tay-Sachs disease	Infection
Down syndrome	Miscarriage
Other disorders	Bleeding

Obstetric conditions

Preeclampsia: presence of protein in the urine, and increased BP during pregnancy. Found in 8% of pregnancies.

Symptoms:	*Tests:*
Abnormal Rapid Weight gain	Proteinuria
Headaches	BP check
Peripheral edema	Weight gain analysis
Nausea	Thrombocytopenia
Anxiety	Evidence of edema
Htn	

Low urination frequency

Treatment:	Induced labor may occur with the following criteria:
Deliver the baby	Eclampsia
Bed rest	HELLP syndrome
Medications	High serum creatinine levels
	Prolonged elevated diastolic blood pressure >100mmHg
	Thrombocytopenia
	Abnormal fetal growth

<u>Eclampsia</u>: seizures occurring during pregnancy, symptoms of pre-eclampsia have worsened. Factors that cause eclampsia vs. pre-eclampsia relatively unknown.

Symptoms:	Tests:
Weight gain sudden	Check liver function tests
Seizures	Check BP
Trauma	Proteinuria presence
Abdominal pain	Apnea
Pre-eclampsia	

Treatment:	Induced labor may occur with the following criteria:
Magnesium sulfate	Eclampsia
Bedrest	HELLP syndrome
BP medications	High serum creatinine levels
	Prolonged elevated diastolic blood pressure >100mmHg
	Thrombocytopenia
	Abnormal fetal growth

<u>Sheehan's syndrome</u>: hypopituitarism caused by uterine hemorrhage during childbirth. The pituitary gland is unable to function due to blood loss.

Symptoms:	Tests:	Treatment:
Amenorrhea	CT scan of Pituitary gland	Hormone therapy
Fatigue	Check pituitary hormone levels	
Unable to breast-feed baby		
Anxiety		
Decreased BP		
Hair loss		

<u>Breast infections/Mastitis</u>: Infection or inflammation due to bacterial infections. (S. aureus).

Symptoms:	Tests:	Treatment:
Fever	Physical examination	Antibiotics
Nipple pain/discharge		Moist heat
Breast pain		Breast pump
Swelling of the breast		

Amniotic fluid

Amnitioic fluid is at its greatest levels at 34 weeks gestation.
Functions:
- Allows normal lung development

- Freedom for movement
- Fetus temperature regulation
- Trauma prevention

Oligohydramnios: Low levels of amniotic fluid that can cause: fetal abnormalities, ruptured membranes and fetus disorders.

Polyhydamnios: High levels of amniotic fluid that can cause: gestational diabetes and congenital defects.
Polyhydaminos Causes:
- Beckwith-Wiedemann syndrome
- Hydrops fetalis
- Multiple fetus development
- Anencephaly
- Esophageal atresia
- Gastroschisis

Gynecological conditions

Atrophic vaginitis- low estrogen levels cause inflammation of the vagina. Most common after menopause.

Symptoms:	*Tests:*	*Treatment:*
Pain with intercourse	Pelvic examination	Hormone therapy
Itching pain		Vaginal lubricant
Vaginal discharge		
Vaginal irritation after intercourse		

Cervicitis: infection, foreign bodies,or chemicals that causes inflammation of the cervix.

Symptoms:	*Tests:*	*Treatment:*
Pain with intercourse	Pelvic examination	Laser therapy
Vaginal discharge	STD tests	Antibiotics/antifungals
Pelvic pain	Pap smear	Cryosurgery
Vaginal pain		

Pelvic inflammatory disease: infection of the fallopian tubes, uterus or ovaries caused by STD's in the majority of cases.

Symptoms:	*Tests:*	*Treatment:*
Vaginal discharge	Pelvic exam	Antibiotics
Fever	Laparoscopy	Surgery
Pain with intercourse	ESR	
Fever	WBC count	
Nausea	Pregnancy test	
Urination painful	Cultures for infection	
LBP		
No menstruation		

Toxic shock syndrome: infection of (S. aureus) that causes organ disorders and shock.

Symptoms:	*Tests:*

Seizures
Headaches
Hypotension
Fatigue
Multiple organ involvement
Fever
Nausea
Vomiting

Check BP
Multiple organ involvement

Treatment:
Dialysis- if kidneys fail
BP medications
IV fluids
Antibiotics

Monitor the patient for:
Kidney failure
Liver failure
Extreme shock
Heart failure

Hirsutism: development of dark areas of hair in women that are uncommon.

Causes:
Cushing's syndrome
Congenital adrenal hyperplasia
Hyperthecosis
PCOS
High Androgen levels
Certain medications

Treatment:
Laser treatment
Birth control medications
Electrolysis
Bleaching

Dysmenorrhea: painful menses.

Symptoms:
Constipation
Nausea
Vomiting
Diarrhea

Tests:
Determine if normal dysmenorhea is occurring.
Pain relief
Anti-inflammatory medications

Endometriosis: abnormal tissue growth outside the uterus.

Symptoms:	*Tests:*	*Treatment:*
Spotting	Pelvic US	Progesterone treatment
Infertility	Laparoscopy	Pain management
LBP	Pelvic exam.	Surgery
Periods (painful)		Hormone treatment
Sexual intercourse painful		Synarel treatment

Stress Incontinence: A laugh, sneeze or activity that causes involuntary urination. Urethral sphincter dysfunction.

Tests:
Rectal exam
X-rays
Pad test
Urine analysis
PVR test

Treatment:
Surgery
Medications
(pseudoephedrine/phenylpropanolamine)/Estrogen
Pelvic floor re-training
Fluid intake changes

Cystoscopy
Pelvic exam

Urge incontinence- urine loss caused by bladder contraction.

Symptoms:	Tests:	Treatment:
Frequent urination	Pelvic exam	Surgery
Abdominal pain/distention	X-rays	Medications:
	Cystoscopy	tolterodine, propatheline, imipramine,
	EMG	tolterodine, terbutaline
	Pad test	Biofeedback training
	Urinary stress test	Kegel strengthening
	PVR test	
	Genital exam-men	

Integumentary System Review

The skin and the specialized organs derived from the skin (hair, nails and glands) form the integumentary system.

Functions

The skin functions by surfacing the body and thus protecting it from dehydration as well as from damage by the elements in the external environment. The skin also helps maintain normal body activities.

Structure

Skin consists of the *epidermis* and *dermis* (*corium*). Deep to the dermis and therefore, the skin, is the *hypodermis*, which is also known as the *subcutaneous* or superficial connective tissue of the body.

Epidermis: The epidermis is derived from the ectoderm and is composed of a keratinized stratified squamous epithelium. *Thick skin* denotes skin with a thicker epidermis which contains more cell layers when compared to *thin skin*. The epidermis ranges in thickness from 0.07 millimeter to 1.4 millimeters. The epidermis consists of specific cell layers:
1. stratum basale or germinativum
2. stratum spinosum
3. stratum granulosum
4. stratum lucidum
5. stratum corneum

Glands

Glands are specialized organs derived from skin. There are two basic types: sebaceous and sweat.
- *Sebaceous Glands*: Sebaceous glands are *simple branched alveolar* (*acinar*) *glands* with a *holocrine* mode of secretion.
- *Sweat Glands:* Sweat is a watery fluid containing ammonia , urea, uric acid and sodium chloride.

- 83 -

There are two types of sweat glands: eccrine and apocrine.

- *Eccrine Sweat Glands:* The *eccrine sweat glands* are simple, coiled tubular glands with a merocrine mode of secretion.
- *Apocrine Sweat Glands:* the *apocrine sweat glands* are very large glands which are thought to have a merocrine mode of secretion.

Hair

Hairs are long, filamentous keratinized structures derived from the epidermis of skin.
Structure: A hair consists of a *shaft* and a *root*.
Hair Follicles: The *hair follicle* consists of two sheaths, the *epithelial root sheath* and the *connective tissue root sheath.*
Hair Growth: Growth of a hair depends on the viability of the epidermal cells of the hair matrix which lie adjacent to the dermal papilla in the hair bulb. The matrix cells abutting the dermal papilla proliferate and give rise to cells which move upward to become part of the specific layers of the hair root and the inner epithelial root sheath.
Hair Musculature: Hairs are oriented at a slight angle to the skin surface and are associated with *arrector pili muscles.* These smooth muscle bundles extend from the dermal root sheath to a dermal papilla. Contraction results in the standing up of the hairs and raising of the skin surrounding the hair.

Nails

Nails are translucent plates of keratinized epithelial cells on the dorsal surface of distal phalanges of fingers and toes.

Wound Care

- Provide a moist environment
- Remove excess exudate but does not allow wound to dry out
- Allows gaseous exchange
- Provides thermal insulation
- Impermeable to microorganisms
- Will not adhere to the wound and cause damage to granulating tissue on removal
- Removal of necrotic tissue is achieved through debridement.
- Debridement options include mechanical, enzymatic, sharp, & autolytic.
- Debridement techniques should be chosen based on desired outcomes, phase of healing, & assessment of advantages vs. disadvantages.
- Common wound etiologies have characteristic presentations that aid in determining etiology.
- Interventions should be based on sound research evidence.
- Wound cleansing can be achieved by various methods.
- Appropriate cleansing techniques are chosen with consideration of the phase of healing.
- Debridement of necrotic tissue can be achieved by mechanical, enzymatic, sharp, or autolytic debridement.
- Wound characteristics need to be taken into account when choosing appropriate dressings.
- Moisture-retentive dressings have many advantages over dry gauze dressings.

Decubitus ulcers:

Stage I: the skin appears red or inflamed. Only the superficial epidermis is involved, though the patient may feel some discomfort. Edema may be present. Stage I ulcers are also termed partial thickness ulcers.

Stage II: the skin appears red, and there may be blisters present. In stage II, the skin has broken. Edema is present, and may extend to the fat layer under the dermis. Stage II ulcers are also considered partial thickness ulcers.

Stage III: the skin lesion reaches the muscle, and there is a thickening of the ulcer's edges. Stage III ulcers are termed full thickness ulcers.

Stage IV: the skin lesion reaches the bone, with possible necrosis of the bone tissue.

Pressure sores can be prevented with frequent weight shifts or turn schedules for patients who are at risk for skin breakdown due to decreased mobility. Care should be taken to position patients so that bony prominences are protected, and shear and friction should be minimal during transfers.

Pressure Points with Positioning

Sitting Pressure Points:
Scapula
Elbows
Sacrum
Ischial Tuberosity
Heels
Greater Trochanter
Popliteal Crease
Toes
Spinous Process

Supine Pressure Points:
Scapula
Occiput
Spinous Process
Sacrum
Elbows
Achilles Tendon
Ischial Tuberosity
Iliac Crest
Plantar aspect of foot
Heels

Prone Pressure Points:
Patella
ASIS region
Chin
Sternum
Forehead
Acromion process
Perianal area

Sidelying Pressure Points:
Thigh
Heels
Knees
Iliac Crest
Elbow
Ear
Toes
Calf
Malleoli
Acromion process

Treatment approaches

Restoration of skills involves remediation of the required performance components such as strength, range of motion, activity tolerance, memory, coordination and fine motor tasks. This approach is appropriate for patients with few skill impairments, or with progressive disorders. Compensation is the next stage and involves teaching the client to perform functional tasks within the limits of his or her performance components. Examples include teaching hemi dressing techniques to a patient after a CVA, or teaching a patient with SCI to use tenodesis for grasp. Adaptation refers to changing the way the task is performed to allow the client to succeed. Examples include providing adaptive dressing equipment, or building up handles on utensils.

OTs generally use a combination of these three approaches in treatment.

Dressing techniques for hemiplegia patients

To don a shirt, a client with hemiplegia should drop the affected limb down into the sleeve of the shirt, and then push the sleeve past the elbow. Next, he should place the stronger arm into its sleeve and use it to pull the shirt over the neck. The shirt should then pulled down in the back with the stronger arm.

To dress the lower body, the affected leg should be crossed over the strong leg. In this position, the patient can more easily reach the affected foot. Pants should be donned over the affected leg first, followed by the stronger side. When the patient stands, care should be taken to ensure pants do not slide down to the floor. To don socks, the patient should cross his legs again, and use his strong hand to hold the sock open and pull it over his heel. He can don shoes in the same position, and should use either Velcro fastens or elastic laces that remain tied.

Positioning Principles

1. Do not use donuts for positioning a wound.
2. Do not use a seat belt in a w/c for pelvic control.
3. Encourage adequate distribution of pressure.
4. Do not substitute egg crates for the proper foam cushion.
5. Wearing the right clothing. Wear clothes that allow the air to circulate and are not too tight.
6. While sitting in a wheelchair, relieve pressure with weight shifts. Weight shifts are done every 20 minutes. Each weight shift must last at least 60 seconds (one full minute) to relieve pressure.

Monitor the patient for:

- <u>Any change</u> in the color of the skin.
- Bruises
- Blisters
- Any opening in the skin.
- Swelling.
- Raised areas
- Hardened areas
- Warm areas felt near a red, dark, raised or hardened area.
- Rashes

Rule of Nines:
Posterior Trunk 18%
Anterior Trunk 18%
Each Arm 9%
Each Leg: 18%
Head/Neck: 9%
Perineum: 1%

Splinting Techniques

When designing a splint, the mechanical considerations should include forces of immobilization, mobilization or stabilization. Care should be taken to ensure the forces do not exceed limits of safety, and that length of the splint is appropriate to the force it provides. The material should be strong enough to provide adequate support, and care should be taken to ensure there is no excessive friction or shear. When constructing the splint, the corners should be rounded and the edges curved to ensure comfort and decreased potential for skin breakdown. All inside edges should be smooth. There should be adequate ventilation for skin integrity, and the straps should be secure and clearly identifiable. When fitting the splint, consideration must be given to the potential for movement within the splint. If the client is able to move too much, the splint may come off or slip to an uncomfortable position. Any structures lying within the splinted area need to be accounted for, such as bony prominences or external hardware.

Splinting the Hand

Safe immobilization of the hand - After an injury, the connective tissues in the hand, such as tendons, ligaments and capsules, are subject to loss of elasticity. This can be caused by disuse, or by the healing process itself. In order to prevent deformities arising from lack of mobility, such as a flexion contracture or claw hand, the hand and wrist should be splinted in a position that discourages shortening of the collateral ligaments. In the "intrinsic plus" or safe immobilization position, the wrist is extended slightly, between 30 and 40 degrees. MCP joints should be placed in flexion, between 70 and 90 degrees, with full finger extension at the DIP and PIP joints. Immobility in this position keeps the intrinsic muscles of the hand intact.

- A dynamic splint is a splint that applies directional force, usually with elastic bands, to encourage passive movement in one plane while allowing active movement in the opposite plain. This encourages gentle elongation of tissues to promote lengthening during healing after an injury such as a tendon rupture. Dynamic splints can also be used to compensate for lack of active movement in one direction during functional tasks. An example of this would be a splint that provides passive finger extension for a patient with radial nerve palsy.

- A static progressive splint provides a constant static force, and is adjusted serially as tissues lengthen. They are often used in cases where contracture is present in order to elongate affected tissues, such as with a patient who has a traumatic brain injury causing severe flexor tone, or with a patient recovering from burns.

Modalities

Ultrasound:

Indications:
Degranulation of mast cells
Thermal US: Increases tissue temperature
Nonthermal US: chemical alterations
Causes release of histamine
Cause fibroblast to secrete collagen
Increase wound contraction
Improve tensile strength of tissue

Contraindications:
Infection
Bleeding
Pregnancy

Electrical Stimulation:

Indications:
Fracture healing
Maintain ROM
Analgesia
Muscle re-education
Scoliosis
Increase blood supply
Stretch Collagen

Contraindications:
Carotid Artery
Pregnancy
Pacemaker
Cardiac Arrhythia

Massage

Indications:
Myalgia
Arthritis
Fibrositis
Scar Tissue
Lymphedema

Contraindications:
Circulatoryt disorder
Abnormal sensation
Metastatic Cancer
Bacterial infection
Bleeding

Thermotherapy is the use of heat to decrease spasms and spasticity in a muscle, or to relax muscles and tendons to increase mobility. Superficial heat can be generated from by heating pad, or by a moist hot pack from a hydrocollator. Paraffin baths may also be used, and generally penetrate subcutaneously. Ultrasound can be set to penetrate heat into deeper tissues. The use of thermotherapy is contraindicated in patients who have impaired sensation, edema, tissue damage, open wounds, cancer or rashes.

Cryotherapy is the use of cold to decrease spasms and spasticity, similar to uses for heat. It can also be used to decrease edema and tissue damage. Cold can be used in the form of an ice pack, ice sticks (used for massage), cold sprays or a cold bath. The use of cryotherapy is contraindicated in patients who have joint stiffness. Some patients may find cryotherapy more difficult to tolerate than thermotherapy.

Effects of ultrasound and iontophoresis

Ultrasound can be used for a thermal effect or a pulsing effect depending on the duty cycle, or continuity of pulse, selected. A continuous duty cycle, or 100%, will provide a thermal effect in order to increase circulation and extensibility in the targeted tissues. This is also a method of controlling pain and muscle spasm. A mechanical effect can be achieved at the pulse rate of 20%, which provides vibration in the tissues to facilitate repair. This can be helpful in the acute phase of healing when heat is often contraindicated, and may increase resolution of scar tissue.

Iontophoresis is a method of delivering ionized medication, often corticosteroids, through the skin and to the tissue using a direct current. It is often used to treat inflammatory conditions, to decrease adhesions from collagen fibers or scars, and to decrease excessive deposits of calcium.

NMES

Before using neuromuscular electrical stimulation on a patient, the OT should assess skin condition and determine if sensation is intact. NMES should not be used if the patient has an absence of sensation, or if the patient has metal hardware under the skin. It is also contraindicated in patients with pacemakers, peripheral vascular disease (PVD), and cancer, and should not be used if the patient is pregnant or has excessive adipose tissue in the treatment site.

Electrodes are placed over the motor point and the opposite end of the muscle belly. The patient should be instructed that he will feel a strong tingle that will cause a muscle contraction. Care should be taken to ensure that the intensity of the current is tolerable. The patient should actively contract the muscle when he feels the sensation of stimulation. After a maximum of 30 minutes, the electrodes should be removed and the skin should be inspected to ensure that it is free from irritation.

Muscular & Skeletal Systems Review

Skeletal System
Axial Skeleton

The axial skeleton consists of 80 bones forming the trunk (spine and thorax) and skull.

Vertebral Column: The main trunk of the body is supported by the spine, or vertebral column, which is composed of 26 bones, some of which are formed by the fusion of a few bones. The vertebral column from superior to inferior consists of 7 cervical (neck), 12 thoracic and 5 lumbar vertebrae, as well as a sacrum, formed by fusion of 5 sacral vertebrae, and a coccyx, formed by fusion of 4 coccygeal vertebrae.

Ribs and Sternum: The axial skeleton also contains 12 pairs of *ribs* attached posteriorly to the thoracic vertebrae and anteriorly either directly or via cartilage to the *sternum* (breastbone). The ribs and sternum form the *thoracic cage*, which protects the heart and lungs. Seven pairs of ribs articulate with the sternum (*fixed ribs*) directly, and three do so via cartilage; the two most inferior pairs do not attach anteriorly and are referred to as *floating ribs*.

Skull: The skull consists of 22 bones fused together to form a rigid structure which houses and protects organs such as the brain, auditory apparatus and eyes. The bones of the skull form the *face* and *cranium* (brain case) and consist of 6 single bones (*occipital, frontal, ethmoid, sphenoid, vomer* and *mandible*) and 8 paired bones (*parietal, temporal, maxillary, palatine, zygomatic, lacrimal, inferior*

- 89 -

concha and *nasal*). The *lower jaw* or *mandible* is the only movable bone of the skull (head); it articulates with the temporal bones.

Other Parts: Other bones considered part of the axial skeleton are the *middle ear bones* (*ossicles*) and the small U-shaped *hyoid bone* that is suspended in a portion of the neck by muscles and ligaments.

Appendicular Skeleton

The *appendicular skeleton* forms the major internal support of the appendages—the *upper* and *lower extremities* (limbs).

Pectoral Girdle and Upper Extremities: The arms are attached to and suspended from the axial skeleton via the *shoulder* (*pectoral*) *girdle*. The latter is composed of two *clavicles* (*collarbones)* and two *scapulae* (*shoulder blades*). The clavicles articulate with the sternum; the two *sternoclavicular joints* are the only sites of articulation between the trunk and upper extremity.

Each upper limb from distal to proximal (closest to the body) consists of hand, wrist, forearm and arm (upper arm). The *hand* consists of 5 *digits* (fingers) and 5 *metacarpal* bones. Each digit is composed of three bones called *phalanges*, except the thumb which has only two bones.

Pelvic Girdle and Lower Extremities: The lower *extremities*, or legs, are attached to the axial skeleton via the *pelvic* or *hip girdle*. Each of the two coxal, or *hip bones* comprising the pelvic girdle is formed by the fusion of three bones—*illium, pubis,* and *ischium*. The coxal bones attach the lower limbs to the trunk by articulating with the sacrum.

THE HUMAN SKELETAL SYSTEM	
Part of the Skeleton	**Number of Bones**
Axial Skeleton	**80**
Skull	22
Ossicles (malleus, incus and stapes)	6
Vertebral column	26
Ribs	24
Sternum	1
Hyoid	1
Appendicular Skeleton	**126**
Upper extremities	64
Lower extremities	62

Characteristics of Bone

Bone is a specialized type of connective tissue consisting of cells (*osteocytes*) embedded in a calcified matrix which gives bone its characteristic hard and rigid nature. Bones are encased by a *periosteum*, a connective tissue sheath. All bone has a central marrow cavity. *Bone marrow* fills the marrow cavity or smaller marrow spaces, depending on the type of bone.

There are two types of bone in the skeleton: *compact bone* and *spongy* (cancellous) bone.
• *Compact Bone. Compact bone* lies within the periosteum, forms the outer region of bones, and appears dense due to its compact organization. The living osteocytes and calcified matrix are

arranged in layers, or *lamellae*. Lamellae may be circularly arranged surrounding a central canal, the *Haversian canal*, which contains small blood vessels.

- *Spongy Bone. Spongy bone* consists of *bars, spicules* or *trabeculae*, which forms a lattice meshwork. Spongy bone is found at the ends of long bones and the inner layer of flat, irregular and short bones. The trabeculae consist of osteocytes embedded in calcified matrix, which in definitive bone has a lamellar nature. The spaces between the trabeculae contain bone marrow.

Bone Cells

The cells of bone are osteocytes, osteoblasts, and osteoclasts. *Osteocytes* are found singly in *lacunae* (spaces) within the calcified matrix and communicate with each other via small canals in the bone known as *canaliculi*. The latter contain osteocyte cell processes. The osteocytes in compact and spongy bone are similar in structure and function.

- *Osteoblasts* are cells which form bone matrix, surrounding themselves with it, and thus are transformed into osteocytes. They arise from undifferentiated cells, such as mesenchymal cells. They are cuboidal cells which line the trabeculae of immature or developing spongy bone.
- *Osteoclasts* are cells found during bone development and remodeling. They are multinucleated cells lying in cavities, *Howship's lacunae*, on the surface of the bone tissue being resorbed. Osteoclasts remove the existing calcified matrix releasing the inorganic or organic components.

Bone Matrix

Matrix of compact and spongy bone consists of collagenous fibers and ground substance which constitute the organic component of bone. Matrix also consists of inorganic material which is about 65% of the dry weight of bone. Approximately 85% of the inorganic component consists of calcium phosphate in a crystalline form (hydroxyapatite crystals). Glycoproteins are the main components of the ground substance.

Changes in Bone

Old Age: Cartilage becomes stiffer and erodes, and bone density decreases. Intervertebral disks become compressed, which can lead to "shrinking" in height. The older adult posture is also more kyphotic with the head pushed forward.

MAJOR TYPES OF HUMAN BONES

Type of Bone	Characteristics	Examples
Long bones	Width less than length	Humerus, radius, ulna, femur, tibia
Short bones	Length and width close to equal in size	Carpal and tarsal bones
Flat bones	Thin flat shape	Scapulae, ribs, sternum, bones of cranium (occipital, frontal, parietal)
Irregular bones	Multifaceted shape	Vertebrae, sphenoid, ethmoid

| Sesamoid | Small bones located in tendons of muscles | --------- |

Scapula

The six scapular movements are: elevation, depression, protraction, retraction, lateral rotation and medial rotation. Elevation is caused by contraction of the upper fibers trapezius and the levator scapulae. Depression is caused by contraction of the lower fibers of the trapezius, and the pectoralis minor. Protraction is caused when the entire serratus anterior contracts, pulling the scapula forward. Retraction occurs when the rhomboid major, rhomboid minor and middle fibers of the trapezius contract. In order for the scapula to rotate laterally, the lower and upper fibers of the trapezius as well as the lower fibers of the serratus anterior must contract. This pulls the glenoid fossa upwards. The pectoralis minor, contracting on its own, will medially rotate the scapula, pulling the glenoid fossa back to neutral.

Joints

The bones of the skeoeton articulate with each other at *joints*, which are variable in structure and function. Some joints are immovable, such as the *sutures* between the bones of the cranium. Others are *slightly movable joints*; examples are the *intervertebral joints* and the *pubic symphysis* (joint between the two pubic bones of the coxal bones).

TYPES OF JOINTS

Joint Type	Characteristic	Example
Ball and socket	Permits all types of movement (abduction, adduction, flexion, extension, circumduction); it is considered a universal joint.	Hips and shoulder joints
Hinge (ginglymus)	Permits motion in one plane only	Elbow and knee, interphalangeal joints
Rotating or pivot	Rotation is only motion permitted	Radius and ulna, atlas and axis (first and second cervical vertebrae)
Plane or gliding	Permits sliding motion	Between tarsal bones and carpal bones
Condylar (condyloid)	Permits motion in two planes which are at right angles to each other (rotation is not possible)	Metacarop-phalangeal joints, temporomandibular

Adjacent bones at a joint are connected by fibrous connective tissue bands known as *ligaments*. They are strong bands which support the joint and may also act to limit the degree of motion occurring at a joint.

Muscular System

Classification

A muscle cell not only has the ability to propagate an action potential along its cell membrane, as does a nerve cell, but also has the internal machinery to give it the unique ability to contract.

Most muscles in the body can be classified as striated muscles in reference to the fact that when observed under a light microscope the muscular tissue has light and dark bands or striations running across it. Although both skeletal and cardiac muscles are striated and therefore have similar structural organizations, they do possess some characteristic functional differences.

In contrast to skeletal muscle, cardiac muscle is a functional syncytium. This means that although anatomically it consists of individual cells the entire mass normally responds as a unit and all of the cells contract together. In addition, cardiac muscle has the property of automaticity which means that the heart initiates its own contraction without the need for motor nerves.

Non-striated muscle consists of multi-unit and unitary (visceral) smooth muscle. Visceral smooth muscle has many of the properties of cardiac muscle. To some extent it acts as a functional syncytium (e.g., areas of intestinal smooth muscle will contract as a unit. Smooth muscle is part of the urinary bladder, uterus, spleen, gallbladder, and numerous other internal organs. It is also the muscle of blood vessels, respiratory tracts, and the iris of the eye.

Skeletal Muscles

In order for the human being to carry out the many intricate movements that must be performed, approximately 650 skeletal muscles of various lengths, shapes, and strength play a part. Each muscle consists of many muscle cells or fibers held together and surrounded by connective tissue that gives functional integrity to the system. Three definite units are commonly referred to:
    (1) endomysium—connective tissue layer enveloping a single fiber;
    (2) perimysium—connective tissue layer enveloping a bundle of fibers;
    (3) epimysium—connective tissue layer enveloping the entire muscle

Muscle Attachment and Function

For coordinated movement to take place, the muscle must attach to either bone or cartilage or, as in the case of the muscles of facial expression, to skin. The portion of a muscle attaching to bone is the tendon. A muscle has two extremities, its origin and its insertion.

Muscle Fibers

A muscle fiber is a single muscle cell. If we look at a section of a fiber we see that it is complete with a cell membrane called the sarcolemma and has several nuclei located just under the sarcolemma—it is multinucleated. Each fiber is composed of numerous cylindrical fibrils running the entire length of the fiber.

- 93 -

Skeletal muscle fibers can be described, on the bases of structure and function, as follows:

- *White (fast) fibers* – contract rapidly; fatigue quickly; energy production is mainly via anaerobic glycolysis; contain relatively few mitochondria; examples are the muscles of the eye.
- *Red (slow) fibers* – contract slowly; fatigue slowly; energy production is mainly via oxidative phosphorylation (aerobic); contain relatively many mitochondria; examples are postural muscles.
- *Intermediate fibers* – have structural and functional qualities between those of white and of red fibers.

Postural support

The erector spinae and the semispinalis are the deep muscles of the back that are responsible for a great deal of trunk movement. The fibers that are arranged vertically extend the spine for erect posture, while the horizontal fibers of these muscles assist with lateral trunk flexion. These two muscles also play a key role in stabilization of the spine during lifting and carrying. The anterior abdominal wall also assists with stability and core strength. These muscles include the rectus abdominis, internal and external obliques, and transverses abdominis. These allow forward trunk flexion, lateral trunk flexion and trunk rotation. Contraction of the abdominals increases the strength and stability of lifting. During walking, the abdominals contract appropriately with each step for maintenance of dynamic stability.

Capsular Pattern

Joint	Capsular Pattern
Temporomandibular	Opening
Occipitoatlanto	Extension & side flexion equally limited
Cervical Spine	Side flexion & rotations equally limited, extension
Glenohumeral	Lateral rotation, abduction, medial rotation
Sternoclavicular	Pain at extreme range of movement
Acromioclavicular	Pain at extreme range of movement
Humeroulnar	Flexion, extension
Radiohumeral	Flexion, extension, supination, pronation
Proximal Radioulnar	Supination, pronation
Distal Radioulnar	Pain at extremes of rotation
Wrist	Flexion & extension equally limited
Trapeziometacarpal	Abduction, extension
MCP and IP	Flexion, extension

Deltoid Muscle

The deltoid muscle has anterior, middle and posterior fibers, which allow for assorted movements depending on whether the fibers are contracted individually or as a group. When all fibers of the deltoid contract, the arm abducts at the shoulder. As the arm returns to the side, all fibers contract to slow its descent. Throughout abduction, the contraction of the anterior and posterior fibers actually prevents forward and backward movement of the arm. When the anterior fibers contract alone, they cause flexion and internal rotation of the shoulder. When the posterior fibers act alone, they cause shoulder extension and external rotation. The deltoid also acts as a shoulder support when the arm carries a heavy load, and is thus frequently involved in scapular and humeral movements.

Brachial Plexus

Commit the following picture to memory. This will probably be on the exam.

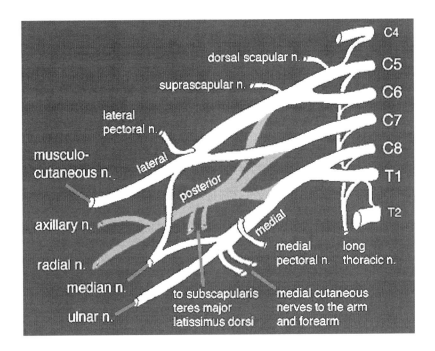

Myofilaments

The thick and thin myofilaments form the contractile machinery of muscle and are made up of proteins. Approximately 54% of all the contractile proteins (by weight) is myosin. The thick myofilament is composed of many myosin molecules oriented tail-end to tail-end at the center with myosin molecules staggered from the center to the myofilament tip. The second major contractile protein is actin. Actin is a globular protein.

Sarcoplasm

The sarcoplasm (cytoplasm of the muscle cell) contains Golgi complexes near the nuclei. Mitochondria are found between the myogibrils and just below the sarcolemma. The myofibrils are surrounded by smooth endoplasmic reticulum (*sarcoplasmic reticulum*) composed of a longitudinally arranged tubular network (*sarcotubules*).

The complex (terminal cistern-T tubule-terminal cistern) formed at this position is known as a *triad*. The T tubules function to bring a wave of depolarization of the sarcolemma into the fiber and thus into intimate relationship with the terminal cisternae.

Contraction

Contraction in a skeletal muscle is triggered by the generation of an action potential in the muscle membrane. Each motor neuron upon entering a skeletal muscle loses its myelin sheath and divides into branches with each branch innervating a single muscle fiber, forming a *neuromuscular junction*. Each fiber normally has one neuromuscular junction which is located near the center of the fiber. A *motor unit* consists of a single motor neuron and all the muscle fibers innervated by it. The *motor end plate* is the specialized part of the muscle fiber's membrane lying under the neuron.

According to the sliding filament theory (Huxley) the sacromere response to excitation involves the sliding of thin and thick myofilaments past one another making and breaking chemical bonds with each other as they go. Neither the thick nor thin myofilaments change in length. If we could imagine observing this contraction under a light microscope we would see the narrowing of the "H" and "I" bands during contraction while the width of the "A" band would remain constant.

Age-related Changes

In the older adult there is a gradual loss of muscle strength, power and endurance as well as general atrophy. Muscles and tendons lose their elasticity, leading to decreased range of motion and a greater the risk of sprains or tears. Cartilage becomes stiffer and erodes, and bone density decreases. Intervertebral disks become compressed, which can lead to "shrinking" in height. The older adult posture is also more kyphotic with the head pushed forward.

Muscle Twitch

A muscle's response to a single maximal stimulus is a *muscle twitch*. The beginning of muscular activity is signaled by the record of the *electrical activity* in the sarcolemma. The *latent period* is the delay between imposition of the stimulus and the development of tension.

Tetanus

When a volley of stimuli is applied to a muscle, each succeeding stimulus may arrive before the muscle can completely relax from the contraction caused by the preceding stimulus. The result is *summation*, an increased strength of contraction. If the frequency of stimulation is very fast, individual contractions fuse and the muscle smoothly and fully contracts. This is a *tetanus*.

Energy Sources

In any phenomenon including muscular contraction the energy input to the system and the energy output from the system are equal. Let us consider first the energy sources for muscular contraction. The immediate energy source for contraction is ATP which can be hydrolyzed by actomyosin to give ADP, P_i, and the energy which is in some way associated with cross-bridge motion.

Special Tests:

Shoulder:

Rotator Cuff Tear: Supraspinatus, Drop Arm Test
Impingement: Hawkin's, Neer's Test, Painful Arc
Biceps Tendinitis: Speed's, Yeargeson's, Ludington's
Lax Capsule: Sulcus sign, Apprehension test
Other Common Tests: AC Jt. Shear Test, Apley's Scratch Test

<u>Elbow:</u>
Tinnel's sign
Pinch Grip Test
Varus/Valgus Test
Wartenberg's Sign
Medial Epicondylitis Test
Lateral Epicondylitis Test
Elbow Flexion Test

<u>Wrist/Hand:</u>
Bunnel-Litter Test
Varus/Valgus Stress Test
Murphy's sign
Hand Volume Test
Finkelstein Test
Tinnel's sign
Allen's Test

Screening

C1/C2	Neck Flexion/Extension
C3/C4	Upper Trap
C5	Shoulder Abduction
C6	Bicep/ Wrist Extension
C7	Triceps/ Wrist Flexion
C8	EPL/ Long Finger Flexors
T1	Interossei
L1-L2	Iliopsoas
L3-L4	Quadriceps
L4	Tib. Anterior
L5	EHL
L4-L5	Heel Walk
L5-S1	Toe Extensors
S1	Ankle Eversion
S1-S2	Planter Flexion
S2	Toe Flexors

Upper Extremity Review

<u>The Wrist and hand</u>
Carpal bones
- Proximal Row
  - ○ Scaphoid
  - ○ Lunate
  - ○ Triquetrum
  - ○ Pisiform
- Distal Row
  - ○ Trapezium
  - ○ Trapezoid
  - ○ Capitate
    - ▪ Head
  - ○ Hamate
    - ▪ Hook of the hamate

<u>Central Compartment</u>
 Palmar aponeurosis
Superficial palmar arterial arch
- Common palmar digital aa.
  - ○ Proper palmar digital aa.
Nerves
    Median n.
        Common palmar digital brs.
        Proper palmar digital brs.

    Ulnar n.
        Common palmar digital brs.
        Proper palmar digital brs.

Flexor m. tendons and tendon sheaths
  - ○ Flexor digitorum superficialis tendons
  - ○ Flexor digitorum profundus tendons

<u>Thenar Compartment</u>
    Muscles
        Abductor pollicis brevis m.
        Flexor pollicis brevis m.
        Opponens pollicis m.
        Tendon of flexor pollicis longus m.

    Nerves and vessels
        Recurrent (motor) br. of median n.
        Superficial palmar br. of radial a.

<u>Hypothenar compartment</u>
    Muscles
        Abductor digiti minimi m.
        Flexor digiti minimi m.
        Opponens digiti minimi m.

    Nerves and vessels
        Ulnar n.
            Superficial br.
            Deep br.
        Superficial br. of the ulnar a.

<u>Interosseous compartment</u>
    Muscles
        Adductor pollicis m.
            Oblique head
            Transverse head
        Interosseous mm. (located between
        the metacarpal bones)
            Palmar (3)
            Dorsal (4)

    Nerves and arteries
        Deep branch of ulnar n.
        Deep palmar arterial arch
            Palmar metacarpal aa.

TAM Score

TAM Score: Finger's Total Active Motion: The total of the extension measurements subtracted from the total of the flexion measurements.

The 10 things that go through the carpal tunnel:
>   4 tendons of FDP
>   4 tendons of FDS
>   Median nerve
>   Tendon of FPL

Anatomical Snuff Box:
>   Anterior boundary - abductor pollicis longus, extensor pollicis brevis
>   Posterior boundary - extensor pollicis longus
>   Radial artery passes through it

Duran flexor tendon protocol

- At surgery, a half (dorsal-blocking) cast is applied with the wrist at 20-30° of flexion, the MCP joints at 70-80° of flexion, and the IP joints straight.
- At 1 week, the cast is removed and a dorsal splint is placed. The wrist is held in 20° of flexion, and the MCP joints are held in relaxed flexion. With the MCP and PIP flexed, the DIP is passively extended. Then, with the DIP and MCP flexed. The PIP is extended. Thus, FDP and FDS repairs diverge.
- After 4.5 weeks, the splint is removed and a wristband with rubber band traction is applied. While awake, the patient passively flexes all joints of the affected finger towards the palm and then actively extends the finger to the splint hood 15-25 times per hour.
- After 5.5 weeks, the patient begins active flexion with wristband removal.
- After 7.5 weeks, the patient begins resisted flexion.

Key Joints		
Joint	*Description*	*Notes*
carpometacarpal joint, finger	the articulation between the distal carpal bones and the proximal ends of the metacarpal bones of the hand	a synovial plane joint; limited motion is permitted at the carpometacarpal joint; the carpometacarpal joint is reinforced by dorsal and palmar ligaments
carpometacarpal joint, thumb	the articulation between the trapezium and the proximal end of the metacarpal bone of the thumb	a synovial saddle sellar joint; this articulation permits two planes of motion: flexion/extension and abduction/adduction which may be combined to produce circumduction
intermetacarpal joint	the articulation between the adjacent sides of the proximal ends of metacarpal bones 2-5	a synovial plane joint; limited motion is possible between at the carpometacarpal joints or between adjacent metacarpal bones
intercarpal joint	joints between adjacent carpal bones	synovial plane joints; small gliding movements are permitted between adjacent carpal bones

interphalangeal joints	the articulations between the proximal and middle phalanges (proximal interphalangeal joint, abbreviated PIP) or the middle and distal phalanges (distal interphalangeal joint, abbreviated DIP)	a synovial hinge joint; these joints are strengthened by medial and lateral collateral ligaments
metacarpophalangeal joint	the articulation between the head of a metacarpal and the base of a proximal phalanx	a synovial condyloid (or ellipsoid) joint; it is strengthened by medial and lateral collateral ligaments; the joint has two planes of motion: flexion/extension and abduction/adduction which may be combined to yield circumduction

Various Grips

Power Grips-Palmar Grips
Cylinder Grasp
Clenched Fist
Hook
Spherical Grasp

Intricate Tasks
Fine Motor Skills (dexterity)
Pinch (Thumb and Finger Grip)
  1. Digital
  2. Tip to Tip
  3. Lateral

Fractures

Chondral fracture	Involves cartilage alone
Osteochondral fracture	Involves cartilage and subjacent bone
Closed (simple) fracture	Skin is intact
Open fracture	Skin is broken
Complete fracture	Involves the entire circumference (tubular bone) or both cortical surfaces (flat bone) of a bone
Incomplete fracture	Break in the cortex does not extend completely through the bone

Comminuted fracture	Involves more than two fracture fragments
Butterfly fragment	Wedge-shaped fracture fragment arising from the shaft of a long bone
Segmental fracture	Fracture lines isolate a segment of the shaft of the tubular bone
Impaction fracture	Occurs when one fragment of bone is driven into an apposing fragment
Depression fracture	An impaction fracture that results when the forces occur between a hard bone surface and a softer surface
Compression fracture	An impaction fracture involving vertebral bodies
Pathologic fracture	Occurs at a site of previous abnormality, often by means of a stress that would not normally cause fracture
Bone bruise	Trabecular microfracture
Stress fracture	Occurs after repeated cyclic loading
Greenstick fracture	Perforates cortex and ramifies in medullary bone
Buckling fracture	Causes buckling of cortex
Bowing fracture	Plastic response to longitudinal compression
Insufficiency fracture	Results from normal stress on a bone with deficient elasticity

Upper Extremity Conditions

Osteoarthritis (OA
Education is very important when treating the patient with OA. OT focus should be on teaching joint protection techniques in order to reduce strain, and work simplification to avoid abnormal postures and wasting energy during self-care and leisure tasks. Typical adaptive equipment for a patient with arthritis is designed to decrease stress on the joints typically affected by the disease, such as the hips, knees, shoulders and hands. A reacher, long handled shoehorn, extended sponge, dressing stick and sock aide will to prevent excessive bending during ADL tasks. Using an elevated toilet seat or lifts under a chair will make sit to stand transfers easier on the joints. Built-up handles for utensils and writing tools are also easier for an arthritic hand to grip.

Rheumatoid arthritis (RA)
The typical rheumatic hand is deviated to the ulnar side at the wrists and the metacarpal phalangeal (MCP) joints. It is also common for the client to have swan-neck or boutonniere deformities in the fingers or the thumb.

It is important the OT review joint protection techniques with the client, not only to reduce overloading the joints, but also to teach compensatory strategies for preventing further ulnar drift. Splinting may be appropriate in order to keep the hands in a functional position for activities, or to prevent contracture. Aggressive ROM is contraindicated due to the inflammatory nature of RA, however gentle passive ROM may be appropriate in order to maintain joint mobility. Use of adaptive equipment can reduce the forces required to complete ADLs, and often items that have larger or longer handles is adequate for joint protection.

In OA, excessive joint loading or repetitive use causes abnormalities in the cartilage or bone of a specific joint. This is usually the knees, hips and hands. Spurs can form in the joints themselves, and pain is a result of decreased shock absorption in the joints during activity. OA generally develops later in life, and is usually a progressive disease.

With RA, a systemic disease affects the joints. Sometimes it can even affect other bodily structures, such as the organs. Pain is caused by inflammation of the joints, and deformities of the affected joints may develop over time. Often the body will feel very stiff. Patients with RA often experience fatigue in addition to their physical symptoms of pain. RA can begin in young adulthood, and is often a progressive disease.

Poor coordination or dexterity
For feeding, a patient can use a weighted or built-up utensil either alone, or combined with a plate guard to ease scooping of food. Sipper cups are also helpful in decreasing spillage. If the patient has a tremor, weights on the wrists can help steady the hands during basic tasks. Patients should not use a razor blade to shave; instead an electric shaver is more appropriate. Garments should be loose fitting, and should have large fastens or elastic bands as opposed to zippers or small fastens. Velcro shoes or elastic shoelaces are useful. Sitting to dress and bathe will be preferable to standing due to involvement of fewer motor groups. Some other useful items for ADLs are soap on a rope, suction cup brushes for nail care, card holders and a large button phone.

Bennet's Fracture
Fracture of 1st Metacarpal
Immobilized: 4wks
Risk of adhesions in web space (maintain positioning)
AROM when cast removed
PROM (6-8 wks) union observed on x-ray
Restore tendon glide
Dynamic Splinting in ROM not gained by 8-10 wks
Strengthening Exs:grasping, fine motor skills, pinch

Carpal Tunnel Syndrome
Median Nerve Compression Syndrome
Loss of sensation, weakness, pain (night)
Splinting - neutral wrist positioning
Modalities: pain & inflammation
Flexibility: wrist & finger flexors, restrict activities, remedy incorrect techniques
Strengthening: wrist, thumb, finger movements
Surgical Procedures: Release of transverse carpal lig.

Cubital tunnel syndrome

Positive Tinel's sign when tapped between the medial epicondyle and the olecranon. Elbow flexion test will produce tingling or jolting sensations.
Aching pain in the forearm.
Poor sensation in both the little finger and the ulnar half of the ring finger.

DeQuervain's Disease
Abductor and Extensor Pollicis Brevis tendons
Repetitive Thumb Abduction & Extension
Spica Splint: slight wrist ext, thumb abd, MCP flex
Splint removed for AROM exs
As pain & edema decrease: strength & end exs
Pinch, wrist & finger, endurance, dexterity exs

Laceration of the Median Nerve
A low-level median nerve laceration affects both the opponens pollicis and the abductor pollicis brevis, causing the thumb to fixed in line with the palm. Contracture may result, as well as wasting of the thenar eminence, resulting in "ape hand". The lumbricals of the index and middle fingers are also affected, potentially causing clawing of these digits. Sensation in these areas will be impaired, as well as fine motor tasks involving thumb opposition and pinch. A high-level median nerve injury also affects the flexor digitorum profundus (FDP) and the flexor digitorum superficialis (FDS).

Laceration of the Ulnar Nerve
If the ulnar nerve is damaged, the intrinsics, lumbricals of the ring and small fingers, and the adductor pollicis (AP) are affected. The result is "claw hand" in which the MCPs are hyper extended and the PIPs are flexed. Sensory loss is on the ulnar side of the hand. Lateral pinch and power grip will also be impaired. A high-level lesion may involve a deep branch of (FDP) as well as the flexor carpi ulnaris (FCU).

Radial nerve compression
Radial nerve compression can cause an inability to fully extend the fingers and thumb at some or all of the MP joints. This is termed posterior interosseous nerve syndrome. There is no sensory loss with radial nerve compression. OT treatment is focused on splinting and PROM to prevent contracture and to maintain function of the hand.

Radial nerve lesion
Radial nerve lesion results in a characteristic wrist drop with an inability to extend the fingers. There is a loss of sensation is on the radial side of the hand, including possible involvement of the medial forearm if the nerve lesion is high. OT treatment is focused on PROM to prevent contracture, and dynamic splinting to maintain hand function. Sensory re-education may be appropriate.

Tendon Injuries:
Flexor Tendons
- Pulley System Present
- Enclosed in Sheaths
- Increase Strength
- Risk of adhesions slightly greater

Extensor Tendons
- No pulley system

- Extrasynovial
- Don't let flexors overpower
- Significant Lengthening required during flexion
- Risk of Adhesions: >impact

Colles Fracture
Dinner fork deformity
Fracture of distal radius with radial deviation of the distal fragment.
Styloid of ulna may be avulsed.

DeQuervain's Syndrome
Pain may radiate into thumb and pain with grasping.
Inflammation of the EPB sheath and APL sheath (synovial lining)
+ Finkelstein's Test

Dupuytran's Contracture
Thickening of the fascia under the palm and fingers.
May initially present as tiny nodules under the skin.
May be noted in children in the thumb.
Causes flexion contractures of the fingers involved.
Surgical intervention is usually required.
OT focus will be on splinting for finger extension, active and passive ROM, scar massage and strengthening.

Mallet Finger
Avulsion of the EPL or EDC tendon from the base DIP joint.

Gamekeeper's Thumb
Rupture of the thumb's ulnar collateral ligament

Boutonniere Deformity
Noted in Patients with RA
PIP flexed, DIP hyperextended

Swan Neck Deformity
Flexion of the DIP and MCP joints
Extension of the PIP joint
Lateral bands slip dorsally at the PIP joint

Medial Epicondylitis
Golfer's Elbow
Medial epicondyle pain

Vokmann's Contracture
Pain with passive extension of fingers
May be caused by supracondylar fx of humerus.
Venous obstruction noted

Complex Regional Pain Syndrome (CRPS)

Caused by vasomotor dysfunction.
Characterized by pain and edema, discoloration and temperature changes.
Sensitive to touch and movement.
OT focus is on pain reduction, AROM and weight bearing activities.

Lateral Epicondylitis
Tennis elbow.
Results from wrist extensor tears at the tendon origin
Due to repetitive forceful motions completed with the wrist flexed.
OT treatment - counterforce elbow strap or wrist splint to decrease load on tendon origin.
Ice, stretching and strengthening are important.

Trigger Finger
Tenosynovitis of the finger flexors due to repetitive forceful grip.
OT treatment involves scar massage to break up collagen deposits.
Tendon gliding through the A1 pulley and work modification to prevent further collagen buildup.

Shoulder subluxation
The humeral head drops partially out of the glenoid fossa of the scapula due to weakness of the musculature in the shoulder girdle. This is common in patients who have had a CVA with hemiparesis, but can also occur after trauma.

Periarthritis
Shoulder pain that is caused by inflammation of the bursa under the acromium or the synovial sheath. It can also be caused by calcification of the rotator cuff tendons.

Frozen shoulder
Results from disuse of the joint, and often occurs after trauma. The shoulder becomes stiff and painful to move, creating a cycle of disuse and discomfort. This causes limitations in range of motion at the shoulder joint, though it usually resolves after the cycle is broken.

Forearm Compartments

Anterior Compartment of the Forearm
Divided into two groups:

Superficial Group-	*Deep Group-*
Flexor Digitorum Superficialis	Flexor Digitorum Profundus
Flexor Carpi Ulnaris	Flexor Pollicis longus
Flexor Carpi Radialis	Pronator Quadratus
Palmaris Longus	
Pronator teres	

Posterior Compartment of the Forearm
Divide into three groups:

Extension and abduct or adduct the hand at the wrist:
     extensor carpi radialis longus, brevis
     extensor carpi ulnaris

Extension of medial four digits
> extensor digitorum
> extensor indicis
> extensor digiti minimi

Extension / Abduction of thumb
> abductor pollicis longus
> extensor pollicis brevis
> extensor pollicis longus

Conditions of the Lower Extremity

Total hip arthroplasty (THA)
There may be a weight bearing status associated with THA depending on the physician's protocol. Until soft tissue has healed following surgery, the patient must avoid hip flexion past 90 degrees, hip adduction past the midline and internal rotation on the operated side. These precautions typically remain in effect for 2-3 months following surgery, though this can vary based on the healing of the joint. A patient who breaks these precautions is at risk for dislocation of the new joint. In order to be independent with ADLs, he should be issued long-handled dressing equipment such as a long shoehorn, extended sponge, sock aid, reacher and dressing stick. Most patients will also benefit from a bedside commode or raised toilet seat to prevent excessive hip flexion caused by sitting on a low surface. A shower stool or tub bench may also be appropriate.

Environmental Concerns

Exercise

Exercise Principles

1. Give verbal cues or directions during exercise.
2. Recognize substitution with abnormal movement.
3. Modify the parameters to fit the activity.
4. Specify your goals from the exercise.
5. Start at the level determined by the evaluation.
6. Base your activities upon your evaluation.
7. Demonstrate the exercise you want to perform.
8. Position the patient in a safe position.
9. Determine the endfeel of the joint.

Muscle Strength Analysis

- 0/5 is scored if there is no contraction or tension in the muscle.
- 1/5 is scored if there is a muscle "twitch" or brief contraction.
- 2/5 is scored if there is active movement through the full ROM in a gravity-eliminated plane. The score is 2-/5 if the movement is less than the full joint ROM, while 2+/5 indicates that the muscle moves the joint through the full ROM, and can take some resistance.
- 3/5 is scored if there is active movement through the full ROM against gravity. If the muscle is only able to move the joint through partial ROM against gravity, the strength is scored 3-/5. If ROM is complete and the muscle can take minimal resistance, the score is 3+/5.
- 4/5 is scored if the muscle is able to move the joint through the full ROM and take a medium amount of resistance.
- 5/5 is scored if the muscle can move through the full ROM and take full resistance, in accordance with age norms.

Types of Exercise

PROM- During PROM, there is no active contraction of the muscle acting on the joint. Because PROM does not strengthen, it should be used only to increase range and to maintain mobility in a joint.
Active-assistive exercise- the patient contracts the muscle and uses this contraction to move the joint through partial range. The remainder of the range is completed by the OT, or with a device such as an arm skate or a mobile arm support. This type of exercise is appropriate to increase strength to allow for full range of motion against gravity.
Isotonic resistive exercise- appropriate when the patient has full range against gravity. Weights or resistance bands may be used to increase strength in the muscles acting on the joint.
Isometric exercise- useful when active range is contraindicated. An isometric contraction is one in which the muscle is activated, but merely holds the joint in position. Isometric exercise can be resistive if force is applied while the contraction is held.

Weight bearing Guidelines

- If a patient has been given the guidelines of using toe touch weight bearing, or TTWB, he is only to use the toes on the affected leg to touch against the floor for balance. This means that during transfers and standing, his weight must be distributed between the non-affected leg and the upper body. Mobility is usually limited, and use of a walker or crutches is necessary.
- With partial weight bearing, or PWB, the patient is allowed to put only a specified amount of weight through the extremity, which can be in the upper or lower body. Weight bearing can be verified during functional with a scale.
- With weight bearing as tolerated, or WBAT, the patient is allowed to put as much weight on the affected extremity he finds comfortable. There are no restrictions, other than what the patient places on himself.
- If weight bearing is full, or FWB, the patient is encouraged to put all of their weight through the affected extremity during activity.

Proprioceptive neuromuscular facilitation

With PNF inhibitory techniques, the OT goal is to decrease tone in a muscle or muscle group, in order to discourage abnormal posturing or positioning. It is also important to decrease the risk of development of contracture through such postures. A method called "hold-relax" may be used to fatigue tight muscles. The patient is instructed to contract the muscle, and hold against the therapist's resistance. Then the patient is instructed to relax, which inhibits the high tone.
Facilitation techniques in PNF include manual contact of the muscle with light brushing, scratching or vibration; stretch stimulus, where the muscle is lengthened as much as possible before the patient is instructed to contract; and activation of stronger proximal muscle groups to excite weaker muscle groups that are distal.

Neurodevelopmental treatment

Methods of inhibiting spasticity in NDT are gentle stretching, reflex-inhibiting patterns (RIPs) through positioning, and weight shifting. Elongation of a muscle with high tone helps to bring balance between the tight muscle and the muscles of the opposing group. Once the muscle has relaxed, the OT can place the limb into a position that inhibits synergistic patterns, usually starting with the proximal motor groups. In addition to positioning with RIPs, the patient can be placed in position to weight shift onto the affected limb, simulating normal movement patterns.

Facilitation in NDT includes joint compression and weight shifting, as well as providing resistance. With weight shifts, there should be a balance between inhibition of the hypertonic muscle and facilitation of the antagonist group. Resistance is often used to encourage muscle contraction in the affected group.

Exercise terms

Kinesthesia: the ability to recognize directional movement in a limb. To test kinesthesia, the OT may ask the client to identify the direction of limb movement without using vision.
Parasthesia: abnormal sensations in the absence of stimuli, such as tingling or pinpricks. Generally patients can report these sensations, however the OT might notice a decrease in ability to discriminate light touch in a patient experiencing parasthesia.
Proprioception: the ability to interpret where a limb is in space, or to interpret the position of the body, based on internal feedback. The OT can test for this by placing one limb into a position in space, and asking the patient to mirror the position with his other limb with his eyes closed.

Stereognosis: the ability to recognize an object purely by tactile sense. This can be assessed by placing common objects into the hand, and asking the patient to identify them without looking.

Akinesia: the patient either does not move the affected limb, or requires a great deal of encouragement to do so. In the absence of instruction, the patient simply leaves the limb unattended.

Hypometria: the patient demonstrates a decrease in the normal intensity of movements. This is often manifested in overshooting objects when reaching for them.

Motor perseveration: the patient does no cease movement in an activity when appropriate. For instance, a patient may continue to move a pencil across paper after he has written his name.

Hypokinesia: similar to akinesia, in that the patient initially may be reluctant to move the limb. Any active movement takes place only after a delay. For instance, a patient who is instructed to pick up a block may require several moments before doing so.

Wheelchair and disability considerations

Adapting to disabilities

In adolescence, a disability causes disruption to the natural cycle of the young adult gradually gaining independence. Due to the nature of an illness or disease, the patient may continue to rely on her parents for basic care needs. This can potentially keep the patient in the role of the dependent child. Adolescents also begin to worry about peer acceptance during this stage. This can be especially difficult for the patient who is "different" due to her disability, and may lead to isolation or lack of adequate social skill development.

During adulthood, making career choices and starting a family are important stages of development. If a patient acquires a disability at this point in life, those roles often require reorganization just as they are becoming natural. She may have to rethink her career and relationships, and the future may suddenly feel uncertain. This patient may be at risk for depression, or self-isolation.

During midlife, a disability disrupts the patient's mastery of his career, and often as his children are entering young adulthood. Just as he learns to balance his roles, a disability causes uncertainty and thus requires reorganization. He may feel as though he is too young to be sick, and may not be ready to allow his children to become his caregivers. This can be more complicated if the patient is the main breadwinner.

In later life, there is a natural expectation of a decline in health. However, this does not necessarily soften the blow of a major disability. Onset of an illness or disease at this stage in life may be harder to cope with due to a frail system. The patient in this situation may fear losing everything they have, or being institutionalized.

Adaptation to a degenerative illness such as rheumatoid arthritis can be difficult, as the course is generally not predictable. Patients may feel uncertain about the future due to in inability to predict relapses and remissions. They may have to be hospitalized frequently. It can be difficult to continually reorganize roles and make lifestyle changes, and patients may begin to lose hope after frequent and progressive losses in ability.

Adaptation to an injury or illness with a rapid onset such as a brain injury can be difficult due to the lack of time to prepare for the situation. A patient is forced to undergo a dramatic and sudden change in lifestyle and roles, and this can be exhausting both to him and to those in his support system. He may feel a loss of identity, and question "why me?"

Wheelchair Seating and Positioning

<u>Seat Base</u>
Contour seating is generally customized to the wheelchair user, and provides specific support to decrease postural abnormalities and to increase alignment. It is also designed to provide pressure relief for patients who are at risk for skin breakdown. The advantage of this system is that it is specific to the individual's needs. Disadvantages include increased difficulty of transfers out of the wheelchair, and greater cost of the product. Also, it must be updated as patients gain or lose weight.

Linear seating is rigid seating that can be custom or factory standard, and is generally more flat with less contours. An advantage of linear seating is that it is generally easier to transfer to and from. Disadvantages are that there is generally less pressure relief, and decreased postural support.

The cushion you select may need to have pressure-relieving qualities and to have a degree of shaping to maintain the pelvic position. The amount of support that is required from the cushion by a patient will vary between patients.

A Jay cushion (J2 or Deep contour) can often be suitable. Pelvic obliquity build-ups and lateral thigh supports can be incorporated within the cushion when required. The cushion must be sized to fit the patient. At the fitting, it is necessary to check that the pelvis is in the 'bowl' of the cushion and that the cushion is not bottoming out.

In cases where substantial lateral thigh supports is required, the supports can be mounted to the wheelchair arm rests or footplate hangar brackets.

A 'dropped' interface board under the cushion can help to stabilize the position of the cushion in the wheelchair and ensure that the patient is not raised up excessively within the wheelchair by the cushion. However, if it is the patient's first chair, it may be best to omit the 'dropped' base in the interest of simplicity.

<u>Back Support</u>
In the young child a preferred posture can often be noted, where he weight bears more heavily through one buttock and where there is also lateral flexion of the neck. In these cases, a firm back support maintaining the lumbar curve can enable the child to sit with a more upright posture.
In these cases, lateral supports should be configured to apply a 3-point support system to the trunk. It is essential that the lateral supports are removable or swing-away to facilitate ease of moving and handling. The backrest is more stable and more adjustable when mounted on the wheelchair with two pairs of arms.

Cases where the patient has a severe fixed scoliosis are becoming fewer due to a multidisciplinary approach in the treatment of these conditions. With such cases the trunk is often best supported with an individually contoured backrest. These should only be used in cases where independent sitting balance is not achievable. A contoured backrest can potentially 'fix' the young person in an undesirable position.

In cases where there has been a spinal fusion, the spinal configuration is largely fixed and cannot be changed by seating. It is possible to provide a more upright posture and improve frontal alignment with the use of a backrest. However it is easy to unbalance these individuals when we change their posture and transverse plane rotations of the pelvic and shoulder girdles can be made worse.

Foot Support

It is important for pressure, deformity and pain management to ensure that the foot is supported along its full length, within the shoe on the wheelchair footplate. The patient should be encouraged to continue using supportive footwear when he is in the wheelchair. Intolerance of footwear is often related to excessive localised pressure. Red marks/callous formation can sometimes be observed on the lateral border of foot. Any footwear tolerance problems should be addressed aggressively and quickly, by ensuring that there is weight bearing in the shoe through the whole foot. Some patients manage to use ankle foot orthoses (AFOs) successfully when in their wheelchair, where as others chose to cease this form of treatment at some stage. To achieve full contact between the shoe and the footplate, it may be necessary to fit angle adjustable footplates and/or extended footplates onto the wheelchair.

Harnessing

The use of a harness within the wheelchair to maintain the position of pelvis on the seat should be encouraged for all patients. If the patient is unable to correct his sitting position when he moves outside his base of support, a chest harness is likely to be helpful. Many patients report that this type of harness prevents them falling forwards when travelling downhill.

Orientation of seating

Ensure the patient is supported in a position where he can function and maintain his posture using the least amount of energy. For the older boys who tend to lean forward, the backrest may have to be reclined by a few degrees and/or a wedge placed under the seat cushion to tilt the patient back a few degrees. This may prevent him from falling forwards and may reduce the need for support through the front of the chest. Many older patients benefit from a powered wheelchair where the seat orientation can be adjusted when required. Tilting back for a few minutes regularly throughout the day may redistribute the loading from under the pelvis onto other areas of the body, relieve muscular-related back pain, and allow the spine to be stretched out from a kyphotic posture that has been gradually adopted during a prolonged period of upright sitting.

Head Support

As the wheelchair is most likely used for work, rest and recreation, the patient who still has a degree of head control may benefit from a head support. Unobtrusive head rests are commercially available. At the stage when the head is too heavy to be supported by the weak musculature a very supportive headrest is required

Arm Support

Armrests may have to be slightly higher than conventionally correct in order to facilitate the use of 'trick' movements. Adjustable-height armrests are often preferred. It may be necessary to add foam 'ladders' to the outside of the arm rest to enable the patient to walk his hand back up the side of the wheelchair after it has fallen off. The arm support should be sufficiently wide to support the forearm, and in line with the control box on a powered wheelchair so the joystick can be accessed. If the patient has no functional movement of the arms, a Velcro strap can help to hold the arms on the arm support in a position where the patient can keep the hand on the joystick.

Ramps

Width: At least 3'6" to give the patient enough space for the width of the wheelchair

Curbing: A low curb (4" high) should be built on each side of the ramp to keep the patient from falling off the edge.

Slope: The incline should not be more than 8%. Federal guidelines dictate there should be one foot in length for every one inch of rise. Minimum width of ramps is 36" inside the side rails.

Turning Space: There should be a level surface at the top and bottom of the ramp. Each platform should be at least 5'0" by 5'0" in size to give the patient enough turning space to move around if they need to.

"Pit Stop" Platform: Plan for a level platform (5'0" x 5'0") for every 30' or so of ramp. This can be changed to fit the patient's needs.

Handrails: Smooth handrails, about 2'6" - 2'8" high, can be built for those who will be propelling the chair by the rails. You also can use them like curbing to protect the patient from falling over the edge.

Ramp Surface: The ramp should be covered with a nonskid surface so the patient won't slide all over the place when it is wet.

Overhead Cover: Whenever possible a cover should be built over the ramp to protect the patient from the elements.

Lighting: Make sure the patient has adequate porch lighting so the patient can see the edges of the ramp.

Entrances

Turning Space: There should be a level surface inside and outside of each entrance. They should be at least 5'0" by 5'0" in size to give the patient enough turning space to move around if they need to.

Threshold: Leave no more than 1, 2" threshold at each entrance. Any more of a threshold will be too big a bump for the patient to pass through the entrance asily.

Doorways

Width: All the doorways in the whole house should be at least 36" wide so the wheelchair can pass through without doing damage to them.

Clearance: There should be a 1' 6" length of clear wall next to the door on the latch side (the edge farthest away from the hinges). This is space for the patient to be out of the way when the door swings open.

Opening Doors: Doors must be able to be opened in a single motion. Remove spring action doors that will work against the patient. To add to the ease of this motion, a door should never be so heavy that it cannot be opened from a sitting position.

Door Handles: The best door handle the patient can have is shaped like a lever. These can be found through some hardware stores, most contractors, and some decorators. This does vary depending on upper extremity deficits.

Bathrooms

Sinks:
- Sinks should be at least 27-34" high.
  Shallow sinks are best (8" deep).
- All exposed pipes should be wrapped to prevent leg burns when hot water passes through them.

Faucet Handles: Faucet handles should be lever type. They should be set back no more than 1' 9" from the front edge of the counter.

Mirrors: Mirrors work best for sitting if they are mounted on the wall tilting downward or no higher than 30" (bottom edge) from the floor.

Knee Space: Adequate knee space below sink that is at least 30" wide and 2'3" high.

Turning Space: Since the turning radius of a wheelchair is a 5' diameter, a clear space of the same size is best in the bathroom.

Fixtures: Ideally, bathroom fixtures (toilet, tub, sink) should be at least 4' apart from one another (if located on the same wall).

Toilet: Generally at a standard height of 1'8". If the patient wants to use an installed shower seat, recommend putting it in about 1 '8" high with grab bars.

Roll-in Shower:

- Doorway to shower should be at least 3'6" and have no curb. Curtain closure or no closure at all is better than a glass or solid door.
- The shower itself should be at least 4' x 4'.
- The floor of the shower should be covered with a non-slip surface.
- Thermostatic controls should be installed in the pipes so that when water is used in other parts of the house (say, a toilet is flushed), the patient won't get scalded. Some parts of the patient's body may not feel the boiling hot water and not signal the patient to get out of the way -- this can lead to serious burns.
- Faucet control, soap holder, handheld shower hose should all be put in at a height that is easy for the patient to reach from sitting.

Kitchen

Ovens & Stoves: Wall-mounted oven and counter-mounted cook top (no more than 2'0" high and with front controls) is best for easy access to the whole appliance.

Counters: Countertops must be no more than 2'6" - 2'10" high. Under them should be knee space at least 3' wide x 2' deep.

Refrigerator: A side by side refrigerator with pull out baskets and shelves works well for people seated in wheelchairs. This gives them more complete access to both the refrigerator and freezer.

Table: Tables in the kitchen should be at least 28 - 29 high from the floor to the underside of its surface so the wheelchair arms can fit under it.

Work Areas: "Work Area" desks are counter tops with side knee space openings (at least 3') are best suited for wheelchair users.

Adaptive feeding equipment

- A plate guard is a curved piece of plastic that slides onto one side of a plate to prevent spillage. It is used to help a patient scoop food.
- A swivel spoon is useful when a patient cannot adequately supinate, to prevent spillage of food before it is brought to the mouth.
- A universal cuff contains a pocket, which can hold an eating utensil, toothbrush or other ADL item with a slim handle. The cuff fits over the hand and secures in place to compensate for weak or absent grasp.
- A weighted utensil has a large, heavy handle and can assist a patient with mild tremors to bring food to his mouth without spillage.
- A rocker knife has a large handle and a curved cutting surface, designed to cut food by rocking as opposed to the typical sawing motion. It is useful for a patient who has difficulty manipulating a standard knife.

Environmental control units (ECUs)

- Level I ECUs include devices that are available for immediate purchase in a store. The device itself will not require modifications to work, though the patient may require adaptive devices in order to make direct selections, such as a mouth stick. They can control basic functions of a few appliances, and on/off switches for lights.
- Level II ECUs include devices that must be purchased from a vendor or manufacturer. They may have adapted switches, and use either direct selection or scanning through selections to control basic functions of several appliances and lights.
- Level III ECUs are also purchased from a vendor, and use adapted switches and scanning. They can control most appliances and lights in the home.
- Level IV ECUs are purchased from a vendor, use adapted switches and scanning, and control most appliances and lights. They are also able to integrate with other systems, such as communication devices.
- Level V ECUs are future technological developments, and are not available to the public.

Safety

Fire Safety:
- Two exits at opposite ends of the home are needed.
- Install smoke detectors.
- An intercom, telephone jack or emergency call system can be placed at the bedside and/or bathroom, or keep a cordless telephone near the patient for emergencies.

Wrapping Pipes: Exposed hot water or drainpipes must be well housed or wrapped with insulated material to protect the patient's legs from bums.

Swing Out Doors: The doors to any confined spaces, such as bathrooms, should SWING OUT. In-swinging doors pose a danger if the patient falls and blocks the door .

Outlets & Light Switches:
- Electric outlets should be placed no more than 4'0" above the floor but at least 1'6".
- Light switches and thermostats should be placed no more than 4'0" above the floor.

Interior Details

The clothing rod in the patient's closet should be set between 3'6" and 4'0" above the floor. This is high enough for most clothing but will still be at an easy reach from the wheelchair.
Shelves should be mounted no higher than 4'6". They should be no deeper than 1'4" so the patient can reach everything. If the patient has a risk of falling, make sure small pets are kept at a distance, and remove any floor rugs.

Special patient considerations

Traumatic Brain Injury Patients
When working with an agitated patient, the environment should be as quiet as possible with few distractions. Clutter should be removed and noise levels should be restricted to a minimum. Structure in the daily schedule and treatment will help to minimize confusion. Before working with the patient, the OT should introduce herself and explain in simple terms what she is going to do with the patient. She should establish easily met goals for the patient, and provide praise or small rewards to positively reinforce appropriate behavior and participation. If possible, she should remove restraints and

Copyright © Mometrix Media. You have been licensed one copy of this document for personal use only. Any other reproduction or redistribution is strictly prohibited. All rights reserved.

position the patient comfortably during treatment. If family is available, she may ask them to bring familiar objects from home to be used in treatment, such as a favorite shirt or a personal hairbrush.

Hearing Impaired Patients

In order to allow phone communication for a client who is deaf or near deaf, a Telecommunications Device for the Deaf (TDD) or fax interface phone is recommended. A client with decreased hearing may benefit from an amplification device. Alarms for fire safety, the doorbell, and alarm clocks should be changed either to a visual signal, such as a flashing light, or a vibratory function. Closed captioning may be appropriate for television if the use of an amplification device does not suffice. Referral to sign language interpreters may be necessary to allow for participation in certain community activities. Finally, local fire and police departments should be contacted, to inform them that a home in their district is occupied by an individual who has a hearing impairment. This information will be useful for authorities in case of an emergency.

OT Administration, Assessment and Management Issues

Assessment of Motor and Process Skills

The AMPS consists of a total of 56 tasks that are rated based on a set number of motor skills and process skills. Tasks vary from sweeping the floor to making a sandwich, and are generally related to performance of IADLs. The client chooses from a selection of tasks that are appropriate to his age and culture in the appropriate environment. Assessment of the AMPS can only be completed by a clinician who has been trained in the AMPS system. Results of this test can predict the client's ability to perform other related ADL and IADL tasks.

As the task is performed, motor and process skills are rated on a 1 to 4 point scale, with1 representing a severe deficit, and 4 representing complete competence.

Functional Independence Measure

The FIM is a uniform data rating designed to rate a client's performance in various aspects of 18 ADL related tasks. It is often used to measure outcomes in clinical settings. Clients are assigned a rating of 1 to 7 in the areas of self-care tasks, cognition, bowel and bladder control, and functional mobility.
A client is rated a 1 if she is completely dependent in a task, or if she performs less than 25% of the activity. A 2 is assigned if she completes between 49% and 25% of the task without help, or requires maximal assistance. She is given a rating of a 3 for moderate assistance, or if she completes 50% to 74% of the task independently. A rating of a 4 indicates that she does at least 75% of the work without help, or requires minimal assistance. A 5 indicates that only supervision or setup is required, and a 6 indicates that she is independent with the task using modifications. Total independence is rated as a 7.

Role Activity Performance Scale

The RAPS is a semi-structured interview for use during evaluation, and was designed to ease treatment planning and measuring outcomes of OT treatment with the adult psychiatric population. It uses a rating scale for the following areas of performance: work, education, household tasks, relationships with loved ones, leisure, hygiene, and ADL performance. Questions that are not relevant are excluded from the evaluation. Answers may be gathered from caregivers or family if the patient is unable to accurately provide information. Each item is rated on a scale of 1 to 6, with 1 being excellent performance, and 6 indicating that the patient is unable to perform the particular task. An advantage of the RAPS is that it can be used to assess progress within particular aspects of the patient's treatment both intermittently, and at the time of discharge.

Canadian Occupational Performance Measure

The COPM is a semi-structured interview that is used to measure the patient's own perceptions of his function in the areas of ADL, leisure, and general productivity. During the interview process, the patient is asked to identify the five most important problems and rate his ability or perceived importance of each on a scale of 1 to 10. A rating of 1 indicates that the patient is not able to complete the task, or is unsatisfied with his performance. A 10 indicates that the patient is able to complete the task very easily, or that he is very satisfied with his performance. At discharge, tasks are rated again, and the difference in numerical values can be used to measure the patient's perception of his own progress, in addition to any changes in the patient's perceived task importance.

Activity analysis

The sensory components that should be considered during task analysis are the abilities to perceive tactile, proprioceptive, vestibular, visual, olfactory, auditory and gustatory stimuli. Perceptually, the following components must be considered: stereognosis, kinesthesia, pain response, body schematics, discrimination, figure-ground differentiation, depth perception, and spatial relations. Clients with deficits in one or more of these areas will require whole tasks, or certain aspects of those tasks, to be graded appropriately.

The motor performance components to be considered for modification during task analysis include fine and gross coordination, range of motion, strength, endurance, postural control and alignment, tone, and praxis.

When grading an activity after task analysis, the OT should consider the most as well as least essential skills required, and adapt accordingly, using remediation as necessary to allow for final task completion.

Theory-focused vs. individual-focused task analysis

In theory-focused task analysis, activities are performed within the theoretical perspective that is being used in the treatment setting. All grading of activity is done within this framework, and changes will be consistent with that particular approach. For example, an OT who is using a behavioral approach with a patient who becomes agitated due to a lack of endurance may address coping strategies. Another OT working within a biomechanical frame of reference may address lack of endurance with remediation of activity tolerance.

In individual-focused task analysis, the client's values and roles guide the OT in adaptations. The treatment focus is on the performance of those activities that fulfill the patient's goals. For example, two patients might lack upper extremity strength, but the OT may work on remediation only with the patient who wishes to carry her child. An elderly client with the same deficit may be independent with her upper body care, and prefer to address a different performance deficit.

Discharge evaluation

Discharge evaluations are useful in determining successful outcomes and can provide important data for evidence-based practice. The purpose of a discharge evaluation is to do the following:
1. Measure progress made since the evaluation date, including number of goals met and number of goals that remain ongoing.
2. Document the final amount of assistance required by the patient for completion of specific ADL and IADL tasks.
3. Update the status of remaining deficits and/or progress in performance components, i.e. range of motion or strength.
4. Make recommendations for the use of adaptive devices or modifications that should be made in the client's discharge environment.
5. Make recommendations for necessary services for the patient after discharge, including ongoing therapy or a certain level of care.

Performance discrepancy

A bottom-up approach to performance discrepancy focuses intervention on the performance components of tasks, using remediation to help the patient reach expected performance levels in self-care. It is thought with this approach that improving the core components of each task will improve performance of the task itself. Examples of OT focus in this approach are strength deficits, abnormal tone, and postural instability.

A top-down approach to performance discrepancy focuses on discrepancies in the tasks directly related to the patient's roles, and the use of generic components for success in those roles. Often, intervention focuses on reducing the demands of the environment so that the patient can function within those roles, using adaptations or modifications as needed. Some examples of this approach are teaching home management tasks from a wheelchair level, and introducing the use of a long handled sponge to wash the back.

Work conditioning and work hardening

Work conditioning involves setting a treatment program based on the basic performance components of a particular employment setting. OT treatment is focused primarily on the deficits that prevent an individual from completing the physical requirements of her job, though it may also include modification of the work environment to compensate for deficits in performance components. Typical interventions are related to deficits in range of motion, strength, coordination and activity tolerance.

Work hardening follows work conditioning. It is a more rigorous program focused on increasing the individual's performance to meet the specific guidelines for a full functional return to her position at work. This is often achieved by practicing work simulations, such as heavy lifting and increasing productive speed in a particular task. Care should be taken to ensure good body mechanics are maintained throughout treatment.

Chronic pain

Clients who have been dealing with chronic pain often have defense mechanisms built up, such as disuse of the affected extremities, abnormal postures or decreased physical activity. One of the first techniques that should be utilized to reduce chronic pain is to involve the client in physical activity. For most patients, this may seem contraindicated. However, it is necessary in order to increase the client's tolerance to physical movement, especially if poor tolerance limits ADL performance. Activity should initially be brief and simple, and gradually increase to a more functional level.
The OT should also focus on methods for dealing with pain positively, such as progressive muscle relaxation, stress management, and distraction. These approaches will help to break the vicious cycle of pain due to nonuse, and nonuse due to pain.

Overt vs. covert pain responses

An overt pain response is what can be seen by an observer, and is usually a behavior. Examples of overt responses are: holding or rubbing the pain site, using abnormal posture or gait patterns to compensate for pain, grimacing during movement of the painful joint and making unusual sounds such as sighing or grunting. A client under observation may be completely unaware that he is exhibiting these behaviors. Conversely, he may also perform such behaviors for attention.

A covert pain response is the internal processing of the pain experience. This cannot be discriminated through observation, and must instead be self-assessed by the client using a rating scale. A client can rate the intensity of pain on a number scale, and describe the experience with words such as burning, or sharp

Motivation and goals

Initially, the OT should select interventions that focus on the individual patient's self-values, especially those that have become more important since the disability began. She should find out what is important to the patient before establishing a treatment plan. Next, she should highlight recent achievements by the patient, and use them as examples to structure future treatments. The OT should share these achievements with the patient and reinforce the actions that are to be admired, such as improving a performance component or meeting a short-term goal. She should also describe the barriers to achieving certain goals, and how these will impede future occupational performance if participation does not increase. If possible, the OT should involve family or individuals whose judgment is important to the patient, so that they may also act as a motivating factor.

All goals established by the OT should be based on the expected outcomes of therapy while taking performance component deficits into account. The long-term goal should be a defined end point of anticipated performance at discharge, and it should reflect the client's resumption of ADL skills within her roles. The short-term goal should be an expected improvement of performance deficits that require remediation for achievement of the long-term goal. Goals should be functional, measurable, and should always refer to the client. An example of a long-term goal is: "The client will complete grooming tasks, while standing at the sink with a walker, with modified independence." The related short-term goal might read: "The client will tolerate 3 minutes of dynamic standing activity, using minimal support, to increase ability with grooming tasks."

Stress management

Successful stress management techniques for chronic stress patients are designed to interrupt the response of the stress reactions of the nervous system, in the same way that interventions for chronic pain might interrupt the body's pain detection system. The goal of OT intervention is to teach the patient coping strategies for dealing with stress. Some of the approaches used are:
1. Aerobic exercise, which can assist in mood regulation.
2. Autosuggestion or mental imagery of sensations of relaxation and warmth.
3. Assertiveness and communication skills training, to decrease misunderstandings.
4. Deep breathing from the diaphragm, to reduce trunk and shoulder tension.
5. Meditation, to decrease or control the parasympathetic response.
6. Progressive muscle relaxation.
7. Time management skills training, to establish order to a hectic schedule.

The OT may use some or all of these techniques with the patient in order to teach him to react more appropriately to stressors, or to avoid the response altogether.

Group vs. individual treatment

In a group setting, patients have the advantage of interacting socially with peers. This can help patients gain social confidence while receiving support from individuals who are going through similar changes. Patients can learn from one other in a group setting, and the OT can be more productive while still providing quality of care. Conversely, group dynamics are more difficult to maintain control over than individual treatments. Also, it may be difficult for the OT to monitor all aspects of the group adequately, which may compromise quality of care.

Individual treatment provides direct one-to-one contact, tailored to the patient's needs. The OT can use this time to work on skills that cannot be completed in a group setting, such as personal care activities. Direct supervision allows the therapist to make any necessary changes immediately. Disadvantages of individual treatment are that there is less opportunity for social interaction, and the patient may feel isolated. It is also less productive for the therapist's time.

Legislative acts

The Americans with Disabilities Act, or ADA, guarantees the same access to state services, employment opportunities, public transportation and housing as Americans without disabilities. It is intended to reduce the difficulty of participation in society of physically or mentally disabled individuals.

The Omnibus Budget Reconciliation Act, or OBRA, was designed to regulate the conditions of long-term care environments in order to increase quality of care for nursing home residents. OT requirements include decreasing the use of restraints, providing comfort positioning, and allowing all residents to have access to activities.

The Individuals with Disability Act, or IDEA, mandates that disabled children should be allowed to receive education in the least restrictive environment possible. It also states that education must prepare disabled children for future independent living as well as employment. The OTs role in the school system, or in pediatric care, is to address this.

Precautions

Standard precautions are those that should be used with every patient, and are designed to reduce the spread of infection. These include the use of gloves when providing direct patient care, as well as washing the hands thoroughly before and after patient contact. As a part of standard precautions, all equipment and surfaces should be cleaned between patients.

Droplet precautions are used when a patient is infected with microorganisms such as influenza and mumps. Patients with droplet precautions should be placed in isolation rooms, and should only be transported if absolutely necessary. In addition to standard precautions, respiratory masks must be worn within several feet of the patient.

Airborne precautions are used when a patient is infected with an illness that can remain in the air for a period of time or over distance. Patients with airborne precautions should be placed in negative pressure isolation rooms and only moved as necessary. In addition to standard precautions, a respiratory mask should be worn by anyone who enters the room.

SOAP note

The "S" portion of the note is the subjective view of the treatment, and should reflect the patient's perspective. It is commonly documented as a quote, such as "It hurts when you move my arm" or "Thank you for teaching me to get my shoes on." The OT should not put her own words here.

The "O" portion of the note is the therapist's objective review of the treatment. It should detail what interventions were administered, how much time was spent in treatment, and what the purpose of the treatment was. The OT should not put subjective material here; only facts should be documented.

The "A" portion of the note is the therapist's skilled assessment of the treatment. Here, she can detail the patient's response to treatment, progress made since evaluation, and expectations for further progress. An example is "the patient was more cooperative today."

The "P" portion of the note details the plan for future treatments. An example is "OT will continue five times per week in order to address deficits in upper body dressing."

Sample Scenarios for OT patients

You are evaluating a patient who has a complete spinal cord injury at the level of C4. Briefly describe his expected functional outcomes, and the OT treatment focus.

A typical C4 tetraplegic will eventually be able to breathe without a vent, though will require some assistance for deep coughing due to lack of innervation of the abdominals and an inability to forcefully exhale. He will be able to elevate his shoulders and will have complete movement of his head. This patient will be dependent in a majority of his self care tasks and will require a lift for transfers. OT focus for this patient will be to train him in the use of a mouth stick for leisure activities such as reading or using the computer. A straw can also be used for this purpose. He will be able to drink from a container that is set up with a straw in reach. This patient will be able to independently operate a wheelchair with an alternative method of steering, such as sip and puff or head controls. Caregiver education is the primary OT focus, however he should also be taught to self-instruct caregivers on his ADL and transfer routine.

You are treating a patient with a traumatic brain injury, who you suspect has left neglect. Describe how you would test for this condition, and list strategies for treatment.

Initial observation of a patient during ADLS can help determine if neglect is present. If the patient leaves food on only one half of his plate, or does not attempt to dress one side of his body, then neglect is likely. Typical evaluations for neglect involve having the patient bisect a line or draw a clock, both of which will be skewed to the attended side.

A patient with neglect must be taught to regularly attend the affected side, and OT treatment should involve participation in activities that encourage crossing the midline. Caregivers should be educated to approach the patient from the affected side to promote environmental scanning. The OT might even arrange the patient's room so that items regularly sought out will be on his affected side. Cues should be provided regularly until the patient is able to compensate appropriately for the visual deficit.

Describe typical deficits and OT treatment for a patient with severe burns in both arms.

A patient with burns is susceptible to decreased ROM due to a rapid rate of collagen formation in the affected area. OTs must perform daily stretching and passive range of motion to decrease the risk for scar band formation. The skin should be moistened with cream, typically cocoa butter, prior to treatment. The stretching should be slow and passive to the point of blanching, or becoming very light in color. Care should be taken not to tear fragile skin, which can increase the risk of infection. The OT may also choose to provide a splint for day or nighttime wear in order to encourage a functional position during healing. The patient should be involved in as many ADL activities as possible to encourage active movement, and caregivers should be educated to follow through with splinting and ROM programs.

A patient enters your clinic with severe edema in her hand. Review some of the possible treatments for her condition, in addition to treatments that are contraindicated.

Appropriate treatments for a patient with edema are as follows:
Contrast baths, which consist of alternately placing the hand in an ice bath and warm water at intervals of a 1:2 ratio, may be combined with active ROM while the hand is submerged.
Compression garments, string wrapping and ace wraps can encourage fluid to move proximally. Care should be taken to ensure the garments or wrappings are not too tight.
Retrograde massage also encourages fluid re-absorption, and involves slow gentle pressure on the affected extremity, applied distally to proximally. Lymph edema massage is a specialized form of fluid mobilization, however performance of this technique requires specialized training.
Finally, active movement combined with limb elevation is an appropriate treatment that can be carried out by the patient and her caregiver outside of the clinic.
Activities which should be avoided when treating edema are direct application of heat, which can encourage further fluid collection due to vasodilatation, and aggressive ROM exercises which can further aggravate inflammatory response.

Describe the OT course of treatment for a patient who has recently had a below the elbow amputation in his dominant arm. He is experiencing hypersensitivity in the affected limb, and has a goal of using a prosthetic limb for functional tasks.

Hypersensitivity and phantom pain are common in the distal stump of recently amputated limbs. In order to prepare this patient for the eventual use of a prosthetic, the stump must be subjected to desensitization. This involves increasing the sensory tolerance at the stump site by progressively introducing textures and increasing amounts of pressure. Examples of this are brushing the site with a towel, or pressing the stump into a cushioned surface. As tolerance increases, the OT should introduce rougher textures and firmer surfaces. Preparation for use of an upper extremity prosthetic should also involve active and passive ROM for maximum joint mobility, and strengthening of the muscles that flex and extend the distal joint. Gross coordination training of the proximal joints is also appropriate. The patient can practice using the stump to push objects around a flat surface, or a paintbrush may be strapped to the affected limb.

You are seeing a patient in the clinic who is undergoing radiation for breast cancer. She presents with decreased ROM in her upper extremities and fatigues quickly during ADLs. Explain why these symptoms are present, and outline the appropriate OT intervention.

In patients undergoing breast cancer treatment, it is common for radiation to have affected the mobility in the joints near the radiation site. Soft tissues in the surrounding areas are often at risk for "radiation fibrosis" which can last for years, even after treatment is complete. Patients with symptoms of decreased ROM and a feeling of stiffness will benefit from mobilization of the affected joints and passive ROM. Heat and ultrasound are contraindicated in patients with cancer, as they can accelerate spread of the tumor cells. Decreased endurance is also common in patients undergoing cancer treatment, and should be addressed through education about energy conservation and work simplification techniques. Providing adaptive equipment to ease the performance of ADLs can assist with these techniques. Examples of appropriate adaptive equipment include but are not limited to a shower chair, a reacher, or bedside commode.

During the initial evaluation, your patient with a complete C6 tetraplegia has established a goal of being able to feed herself independently, with the least amount of equipment possible.

Currently, she is has 3/5 strength for shoulder flexion, and 3+/5 for elbow flexion. Finger flexion is absent. Describe the stages of progressing this patient to her goal.

The initial OT focus should be strength and endurance of shoulder flexion, to ensure hand to mouth movements can be sustained for the duration of the feeding task. If the patient fatigues quickly, she may be initially provided with a mobile arm support to assist in feeding. In the absence if finger flexion, a universal cuff can allow her to hold a utensil, using a plate guard as a barrier for spill-free scooping. A cup with a large handle or a long straw can be provided to ease drinking. As shoulder strength progresses, the mobile arm support should be discontinued. The OT should also focus on increasing the strength of tenodesis grasp in order to allow the patient to hold a utensil without a cuff. A built-up handle for the utensil may be necessary initially or permanently. In order to make eating more efficient, the OT should focus on strengthening the specific movements that ease scooping or stabbing food, bringing the hand to the mouth and releasing the hand after biting.

Describe the differences between the typical behaviors of a patient who is at an Allen Cognitive Level of 2.4-2.8 versus a patient who is 3.8-4.0.

In Allen level 2.4-2.8, or late dementia, patients still have the gross motors skills required to walk. They tend to wander, or participate in repetitive motions like rocking. In general, they are not able to perform appropriate actions on objects such as articles of clothing. They can respond to simple cues related to movement, such as instruction to stand up after toileting. Usually patients at this level can feed themselves finger foods and self-administer beverages.
At level 3.8-4.0, or early dementia, patients can complete basic self-care skills in a routine. They have deficits in problem solving, and are unable to get past roadblocks in their basic routines. For instance, a patient who runs out of toilet paper might attempt to clean himself with his hand. Patients at this level cannot be reasoned with, and may become agitated if given too much information to process. They are able to learn new skills with repetition.

You are treating a patient on a dementia unit who is at Allen Cognitive Level 4.4. Her caregiver states that she was able to complete her ADLs at home, however she has been dependent since her admission to the unit. List several strategies that might increase this patient's involvement in her personal care.

One of the first things the therapist should do is to find out the patient's former ADL routine from the caregiver, including start time, time needed to complete, and basic setup at home. Next, the therapist should simulate these conditions as closely as possible to maximize the patient's involvement. Some strategies that might encourage greater participation include placing all ADL items in plain view at eye level in the area where they will be used. Clothing choices should be minimized, or pre-arranged outfits should be set out for the patient. Also, extra time should be allowed for this patient to complete her routine. Once an appropriate routine is established, the therapist should ensure that caregivers on the unit are educated regarding the patient's ADL abilities.

A patient in his thirties is refusing treatment, stating that his wife will dress him at home. His wife works full-time, and he does not qualify for homecare assistance. The patient appears to be depressed. Describe what approach the OT should take to encourage participation.

A patient who appears to be depressed should be referred to a counselor or social worker, and a description of his mood and actions should be passed along to the treating nurses and physicians. In order to encourage the patient to participate, the OT should explain the reasoning behind the treatment she is providing. She should never try to force the patient to do something he does not want to do; however, she should try to find a common ground with him. The next step should be to establish goals with the patient, to determine what is important to him. A patient who is working towards his own personal goal will be more likely to participate that a patient whose established goal does not inspire him. Once the patient is cooperating more, the therapist should set several goals that are quickly achievable. The patient should be reminded of his progress, and mood should be monitored for changes.

Give examples of how to make the task of preparing a sandwich simpler or more demanding on a patient's physical and cognitive abilities.

To grade thus task so that it will be easier for the client physically, the OT can do any of the following things: place ingredients on a shelf within reach, use adaptive devices such as a built-up knife or jar opener, allow the patient to sit, move items closer to the patient, allow the patient to take breaks, or remove appropriate items from packaging. Cognitively, the OT can reduce the number of ingredient choices, provide instruction during each step, cue for location of items, provide a checklist, or allow extra time for completion of the task

To grade the activity so that it is more difficult physically, the OT might have the patient stand, retrieve the ingredients from various locations, open containers and packaging without assistance, or complete within an allotted time frame. To make it more challenging cognitively, she may ask the patient to complete the task without instruction, or provide multi-step cues and directions. The OT can also ask the patient to locate the ingredients, and to recall safety without cues.

You are treating a patient with MS whose main goal is to shower in her bathtub with minimal assistance. Currently, she can tolerate 5 minutes of activity at a time and requires moderate assistance to stand and transfer. Describe OT intervention, including use of adaptive devices.

Due to the relapsing and remitting nature of MS, it is important that her therapy and any adaptive equipment provided be appropriate for various levels of the patient's abilities. The first step in OT treatment is to increase her activity tolerance so that a shower will not exhaust her. The patient should participate in endurance training, and dynamic upper body tasks in order to increase tolerance to a more functional level. Next, she should be educated on energy conservation and work simplification. To make showering easier, she can use a tub transfer bench, a long sponge and a handheld shower. The OT should provide training on the use of these items. Caregiver education is also important, as the patient plans to receive some assistance at home. Finally, the OT should complete transfer training and standing tolerance activities to increase the patient's ability with shower transfers, and standing briefly for hygiene.

You are evaluating a patient with an incomplete spinal cord injury (SCI) at the level C7. Describe manual muscle and sensory testing for this patient, including variations to be expected from a patient with a complete injury at the same level.

When completing a sensory or motor test with a patient who has SCI, the patient should be in supine in bed or on a mat, wearing non-restrictive clothing. This will enable the OT to fully access the upper extremities, and to perform both gravity-eliminated and against gravity measurements of muscle strength. The patient's sensation should be measured for deficits in the detection of light touch and pain (a pin prick) in accordance with dermatomes.

- 124 -

A patient with an SCI at C7, who has no other upper extremity injuries, would be expected to have at least fair strength in biceps, triceps, wrist extensors and finger flexors. Sensation should be intact to the C7 dermatome on the lateral forearm. A patient with an incomplete injury may have deficits in sensation and strength at the site of injury, however areas tested below the injury may be partially intact on one or both sides of the body.

You are working with a client who has right hemiparesis. He is able to stand with supervision using a bar for support, and is independent with wheelchair mobility. He can tolerate 20 minutes of activity before needing to rest. He lives with his wife, who can provide limited physical assistance at home. His goal is to be as independent as possible with his self-care. Describe the adaptive equipment that would be appropriate for this patient.

The patient should go home at a wheelchair level for safety, and thus a lightweight wheelchair should be provided to allow for easy car transport for outings and doctor's appointments. Grooming skills can be performed at the sink from the wheelchair. A suction brush may be appropriate for nail care. The patient may benefit from the use of a reacher during dressing tasks, and to safely access fallen items. A long shoehorn and a dressing stick can decrease the demands of dressing tasks, as can the use of Velcro, elastic shoelaces, and a button hook. A raised toilet seat and a shower chair in conjunction with installation of grab bars are recommended for the bathroom. The patient will also benefit from a handheld shower, as well as long sponge to ease washing of the non-affected extremity. Non-slip surfaces should be used in the shower and on the bathroom floor to decrease the risk of falls.

You are treating an elderly patient in a sub acute care setting who has suffered a severe CVA. He has reached a plateau, and requires moderate to maximal assistance with his ADLs and transfers. His wife says she would like to take him home. Describe the next appropriate steps to take in your treatment.

This patient will require a great deal of physical help at home, and may require even more help when he is fatigued at the end of the day. Maintaining this level of physical activity is taxing on a caregiver, especially an elderly female. The first step for the OT should be to provide direct family training in all aspects of the patient's self care needs. The spouse should begin to assist with the patient's dressing and bathing, toileting tasks and transfers. The OT's role is to determine whether she is able to safety care for the patient. The next step is to refer the patient to the social worker, who provide advise about community resources to ease the caregiver burden, such as a bath aide. The social worker can also discuss other options for care, and provide any necessary counseling. Often, elderly spouses feel a strong sense of responsibility to care for their loved ones, but it is up to the team to determine whether or not this will meet the patient's needs.

Special Report: NBCOT Sample Questions

1. An occupational therapist is working in an outpatient orthopedic clinic. During the patient's history the patient reports, "I tore 3 of my 4 Rotator cuff muscles in the past." Which of the following muscles cannot be considered as possibly being torn?
A: Teres minor
B: Teres major
C: Supraspinatus
D: Infraspinatus

2. An occupational therapist at an outpatient clinic is returning phone calls that have been made to the clinic. Which of the following calls should have the highest priority for medical intervention?
A: A home health patient reports, "I am starting to have breakdown of my heels."
B: A patient that received an upper extremity cast yesterday reports, "I can't feel my fingers in my right hand today."
C: A young female reports, "I think I sprained my ankle about 2 weeks ago."
D: A middle-aged patient reports, "My knee is still hurting from the TKR."

3. An occupational therapist is assessing a rupture of the ulnar collateral ligament of the thumb. Which of the following terms is another phrase for this condition?
A: Mallet finger
B: Gamekeeper's thumb.
C: Herberden's nodes
D: Early signs of CTS.

4. An occupational therapist is performing a screening on a patient that has been casted recently on the left upper extremity. Which of the following statements should the occupational therapist be most concerned about?
A: The patient reports, "I didn't keep my extremity elevated like the doctor asked me to."
B: The patient reports, "I have been having pain in my left forearm."
C: The patient reports, "My left arm has really been itching."
D: The patient reports, "The arthritis in my wrists is flaring up, when I put weight on my crutch."

5. A 93 year-old female with a history of Alzheimer's Disease gets admitted to an Alzheimer's unit. The patient has exhibited signs of increased confusion and limited stability with gait. Moreover, the patient is refusing to use a w/c. Which of the following is the most appropriate course of action for the occupational therapist?
A: Recommend the patient remain in her room at all times.
B: Recommend family members bring pictures to the patient's room.
C: Recommend a speech therapy consult to the doctor.
D: Recommend the patient attempt to walk pushing the w/c for safety.

6. An occupational therapist is covering a pediatric unit and is responsible for a 15 year-old male patient on the floor. The mother of the child states, "I think my son is sexually interested in girls." The most appropriate course of action of the occupational therapist is to respond by stating:
A: "I will talk to the doctor about it."
B: "Has this been going on for a while?"

C: "How do you know this?"
D: "Teenagers often exhibit signs of sexual interest in females."

7. An occupational therapist is caring for a patient who has recently been diagnosed with fibromyalgia and COPD. Which of the following tasks should the occupational therapist delegate to an aide?
A: Transferring the patient during the third visit.
B: Evaluating the patient
C: Taking the patient's vital sign while setting up an exercise program
D: Educating the patient on monitoring fatigue

8. An occupational therapist has been instructed to provide hand wound care for a patient that has active TB and HIV. The occupational therapist should where which of the following safety equipment?
A: Sterile gloves, mask, and goggles
B: Surgical cap, gloves, mask, and proper shoewear
C: Double gloves, gown, and mask
D: Goggles, mask, gloves, and gown

9. Which of the following correctly identifies the TAM score?
A: The total of a finger's flexion measurements minus the total extension measurements.
B: The total of a finger's extension measurements minus the total flexion measurements.
C: The total of a finger's flexion measurements minus the total extension measurements divided by 2.
D: The total of a finger's extension measurements minus the total flexion measurements divided by 2.

10. A 64 year-old Alzheimer's patient has exhibited excessive cognitive decline resulting in harmful behaviors. The physician orders restraints to be placed on the patient. Which of the following is the appropriate procedure?
A: Secure the restraints to the bed rails on all extremities.
B: Notify the physician that restraints have been placed properly.
C: Communicate with the patient and family the need for restraints.
D: Position the head of the bed at a 45 degree angle.

11. A 22 year-old patient in a mental health lock-down unit under suicide watch appears happy about being discharged. Which of the following is probably happening?
A: The patient is excited about being around family again.
B: The patient's suicide plan has probably progressed.
C: The patient's plans for the future have been clarified.
D: The patient's mood is improving.

12. A patient that has delivered a 8.2 lb. baby boy 3 days ago via c-section, reports white patches on her breast that aren't going away. Which of the following medications may be necessary?
A: Nystatin
B: Atropine
C: Amoxil
D: Loritab

13. A 64 year-old male who has been diagnosed with COPD, and CHF. The patient exhibits an increase in total body weight of 10 lbs. over the last few days during inpatient therapy. The occupational therapist should:
A: Contact the patient's physician immediately.

- 127 -

B: Check the intake and output on the patient's flow sheet.

C: Encourage the patient to ambulate to reduce lower extremity edema.

D: Check the patient's vitals every 2 hours.

14. A patient that has TB can be taken off restrictions after which of the following parameters have been met?

A: Negative culture results.

B: After 30 days of isolation.

C: Normal body temperature for 48 hours.

D: Non-productive cough for 72 hours.

15. An occupational therapist teaching a patient with COPD pulmonary exercises should do which of the following?

A: Teach purse-lip breathing techniques.

B: Encourage repetitive heavy lifting exercises that will increase strength.

C: Limit exercises based on respiratory acidosis.

D: Take breaks every 10-20 minutes with exercises.

16. A patient asks an occupational therapist the following question. Exposure to TB can be identified best with which of the following procedures?

A: Chest x-ray

B: Mantoux test

C: Breath sounds examination

D: Sputum culture for gram-negative bacteria

17. A twenty-one year old man suffered a concussion during therapy and the MD ordered a MRI. The patient asks, "Will they allow me to sit up during the MRI?" The correct response by the occupational therapist should be.

A: "I will have to talk to the doctor about letting you sit upright during the test."

B: "You will be positioned in the reverse Trendelenburg position to maximize the view of the brain."

C: "The radiologist will let you know."

D: "You will have to lie down on your back during the test."

18. A fifty-five year-old man suffered a left frontal lobe CVA. Which of the following should the occupational therapist watch most closely for?

A: Changes in emotion and behavior

B: Monitor loss of hearing

C: Observe appetite and vision deficits

D: Changes in facial muscle control

19. An occupational therapist working in a pediatric clinic observes bruises on the body of a four year-old boy. The parents report the boy fell riding his bike. The bruises are located on his posterior chest wall and gluteal region. The occupational therapist should:

A: Suggest a script for counseling for the family to the doctor on duty.

B: Recommend a warm bath for the boy to decrease healing time.

C: Notify the case manager in the clinic about possible child abuse concerns.

D: Recommend ROM to the patient's spine to decrease healing time.

20. A 14 year-old boy has been admitted to a mental health unit for observation and treatment for a broken wrist and shoulder. The boy becomes agitated and starts yelling at staff members. What should the occupational therapist first response be?
A: Create an atmosphere of seclusion for the boy according to procedures.
B: Remove other patients from the area via wheelchairs for added speed.
C: Ask the patient, "What is making you mad?"
D: Ask the patient, "Why are you doing this, have you thought about what your parents might say?"

21. An occupational therapist is instructing a patient on the order of sensations with the application of an ice water bath for a swollen L wrist. Which of the following is the correct order of sensations experienced with an ice water bath?
A: cold, burning, aching, and numbness
B: burning, aching, cold, and numbness
C: aching, cold, burning and numbness
D: cold, aching, burning and numbness

22. An occupational therapist wants to test a patient's ability to sweat. Which of the following assessment tools or techniques would be used?
A: heated whirlpool
B: ninhydrin test
C: tuning fork
D: counter hydration test

23. An occupational therapist assesses a 43 year carpenter that has recently broken 70% of the bones in his right upper extremity. The carpenter is insistent upon returning to work at the end of the week and being cleared by OT for full duties. Which of the following categories would the patient be placed in on the disability adjustment stage?
A: Acceptance
B: Grieving
C: Anger
D: Denial

24. Tricyclics (Antidepressants) sometimes have which of the following adverse affects on patients that have a diagnosis of depression?
A: Shortness of breath
B: Fainting
C: Large Intestine ulcers
D: Distal muscular weakness

25. An occupational therapist is instructing a patient about the warning signs of (Digitalis) side effects. Which of the following side effects should the occupational therapist tell the patient are sometimes associated with excessive levels of Digitalis?
A: Seizures
B: Muscle weakness
C: Depression
D: Anxiety

26. An occupational therapist is assessing a patient in an acute care setting. The patient has the following signs: weak pulse, quick respiration, acetone breath, and nausea. Which of the following conditions is most likely occurring?
A: Hypoglycemic patient
B: Hyperglycemic patient
C: Cardiac arrest
D: End-stage renal failure

27. Medical records indicate a patient has developed a condition of respiratory alkalosis. Which of the following clinical signs would not apply to a condition of respiratory alkalosis?
A: Muscle tetany
B: Syncope
C: Numbness
D: Anxiety

28. Which of the following lab values would indicate symptomatic AIDS in the medical chart? (T4 cell count per deciliter)
A: Greater than 1000 cells per deciliter
B: Less than 500 cells per deciliter
C: Greater than 2000 cells per deciliter
D: Less than 200 cells per deciliter

29. An occupational therapist is assessing a patient that has undergone a recent CABG. The occupational therapist notices a mole with irregular edges with a bluish color. The occupational therapist should:
A: Recommend a dermatological consult to the MD.
B: Note the location of the mole and contact the physician via the telephone.
C: Note the location of the mole and follow-up with the attending physician via the medical record and phone call.
D: Remove the mole with a sharp's debridement technique.

30. An occupational therapist is assessing a 18 year-old female who has recently suffered a TBI. The occupational therapist notes a slower pulse and impaired respiration. The occupational therapist should report these findings immediately to the physician, due to the possibility the patient is experiencing which of the following conditions?
A: Increased intracranial pressure
B: Increased function of cranial nerve X
C: Sympathetic response to activity
D: Meningitis

31. An occupational therapist is making discharge recommendations to patient that has recently been diagnosed with COPD, Arthritis, and an Anxiety disorder. Which of the following recommendations would be the most helpful for the patient to take their medicine correctly?
A: A chart that will have the pills and times broken down in the bathroom.
B: A pill container that has different time slots.
C: A brightly colored pill container to avoid getting lost.
D: Easy access tops on the medication and large labels on the containers.

32. An occupational therapist has been assigned a patient who has recently been diagnosed with Guillain-Barre' Syndrome. Which of the following statements is the most applicable when discussing the impairments with Guillain-Barre' Syndrome with the patient?
A: Guillain-Barre' Syndrome gets better after 5 years in almost all cases.
B: Guillain-Barre' Syndrome causes limited sensation in the abdominal region.
C: Guillain-Barre' Syndrome causes muscle weakness in the legs.
D: Guillain-Barre' Syndrome does not effect breathing in severe cases.

33. An occupational therapist is returning phone calls in a pediatric clinic. Which of the following reports most requires the occupational therapist's immediate attention and phone call?
A: A 8 year-old boy has been vomiting and appears to have slower movements and has a history of an atrio-ventricular shunt placement.
B: A 10 year-old girl feels a dull pain in her abdomen after doing sit-ups in gym class.
C: A 7 year-old boy has been having a low fever and headache for the past 3 days that has history of an anterior hand wound.
D: A 7 year-old girl that had a cast on her right wrist is complaining of itching.

34. An occupational therapist is assessing a patient in the rehab unit. The patient has suffered a TBI 3 weeks ago. Which of the following is the most distinguishing characteristic of a neurological disturbance?
A: LOC (level of consciousness)
B: Short term memory
C: + Babinski sign
D: + Clonus sign

35. A patient is currently having a petit mal seizure in the clinic on the floor. Which of the following criteria has the highest priority in this situation?
A: Provide a safe environment free of obstructions in the immediate area
B: Call a code
C: Contact the patient's physician
D: Prevent excessive movement of the extremities

36. An occupational therapist is caring for a patient in the step down unit. The patient has signs of increased intracranial pressure. Which of the following is not a sign of increased intracranial pressure?
A: Bradycardia
B: Increased pupil size bilaterally
C: Change in LOC
D: Vomiting

37. The charge nurse on a cardiac unit tells you a patient is exhibiting signs of right-sided heart failure. Which of the following would not indicate right-sided heart failure?
A: Nausea
B: Anorexia
C: Rapid weight gain
D: SOB (shortness of breath)

38. A 24 year-old man has been admitted to the hospital due to work-related injury. The patient's wife would like to see the patient's chart. The occupational therapist should:
A: Provide the chart to the patient's wife following verbal approval by the patient.

B: Provide the chart to the patient's wife after consulting with the patient's physician.
C: Get written approval from the patient prior to providing the wife with chart information and call the MD about the patient's request.
D: Tell the patient' wife, a copy of the patient's medical record is on-file with medical records.

39. A 49 year old female is in rehab for a TBI. Which of the following home tasks would take the greatest amount of problem solving and should be practiced in rehab?
A: Reading a book for pleasure.
B: Practice finding small objects like: car keys.
C: Grooming and self-care ADLs.
D: Preparing a simple meal.

40. A patient has just been prescribed Minipress to control hypertension. The occupational therapist should instruct the patient to be observant of the following:
A: Dizziness and light headed sensations
B: Weight gain
C: Sensory changes in the lower extremities
D: Fatigue

41. An occupational therapist is performing an evaluation on patient's wrist. Which of the following diagnostic terms matches the following information: Extension noted at the PIP joint, Flexion of the MCP and DIP joints. Lateral bands have slipped dorsally at the PIP joint?
A: Mallet finger
B: Swan Neck deformity
C: Boutonniere's deformity
D: Claw fingers

42. A 55 year-old female asks an occupational therapist the following, "Which mineral/vitamin is the most important to prevent progression of osteoporosis. The occupational therapist should state:
A: Potassium
B: Magnesium
C: Calcium
D: Vitamin B12

43. A patient has recently been diagnosed with symptomatic bradycardia. Which of the following medications is the most recognized for treatment of symptomatic bradycardia?
A: Questran
B: Digitalis
C: Nitroglycerin
D: Atropine

44. A patient has recently been prescribed Lidocaine Hydrochloride. Which of the following symptoms may occur with over dosage?
A: Memory loss and lack of appetite
B: Confusion and fatigue
C: Heightened reflexes
D: Tinnitus and spasticity

45. Which of the following recommendations would be the most helpful for someone who has right hemiplegia and is going to a driving program offered by occupational therapy?
A: Variable digital and voice controls
B: Alternate brake position
C: Hand controls with stick on the L
D: Use of a spinner knob to aid with steering

46. A patient has suffered a left CVA and has developed severe hemiparesis resulting in a loss of mobility. The occupational therapist notices on assessment that an area over the patient's left elbow appears as non-blanchable erythema and the skin is intact. The occupational therapist should score the patient as having which of the following?
A: Stage I pressure ulcer
B: Stage II pressure ulcer
C: Stage III pressure ulcer
D: Stage IV pressure ulcer

47. A newborn baby exhibits a reflex that includes: hand opening, abducted and extended extremities following a jarring motion. Which of the following correctly identifies the reflex?
A: ATNR reflex
B: Startle reflex
C: Grasping reflex
D: Moro reflex

48. An occupational therapist suspects a patient is developing Bell's Palsy. The occupational therapist wants to test the function of cranial nerve VII. Which of the following would be the most appropriate testing procedures?
A: Test the taste sensation over the back of the tongue and activation of the facial muscles.
B: Test the taste sensation over the front of the tongue and activation of the facial muscles.
C: Test the sensation of the facial muscles and sensation of the back of the tongue.
D: Test the sensation of the facial muscles and sensation of the front of the tongue.

49. An occupational therapist is reviewing a patient's serum glucose levels. Which of the following scenarios would indicate abnormal serum glucose values for a 30 year-old male?
A: 70 mg/dl
B: 55 mg/dl
C: 110 mg/dl
D: 100 mg/dl

50. A two-year old has been in the hospital for 3 weeks and seldom seen family members due to isolation precautions. Which of the following hospitalization changes is most like to be occurring?
A: Guilt
B: Trust
C: Separation anxiety
D: Shame

51. An occupational therapist is working in a pediatric clinic and a 25 year-old mother comes in with a 12 week-old baby for initial evaluation. The mother is stress out about loss of sleep and the baby exhibits signs of colic. Which of the following techniques should the occupational therapist teach the mother?

- 133 -

A: Distraction of the infant with a red object
B: Prone positioning techniques
C: Tapping reflex techniques
D: Neural warmth techniques

52. An occupational therapist is working in a pediatric clinic and a mother brings in her 13 month old child who has Down Syndrome. The mother reports, "My child's muscles feel weak and he isn't moving well. My RN friend check his reflexes and she said they are diminished." Which of the following actions should the occupational therapist take first?
A: Contact the physician immediately
B: Have the patient go to X-ray for a c-spine work-up.
C: Start an IV on the patient
D: Position the child's neck in a neutral position

53. An occupational therapist is evaluating a child's voluntary release of a toy? Complete release that is voluntary should occur by?
A: 6 months
B: 8 months
C: 10 months
D: 12 months

54. A 29 year-old male has a diagnosis of AIDS. The patient has had a two year history of AIDS. The most like cognitive deficits include which of the following?
A: Disorientation
B: Sensory changes
C: Inability to produce sound
D: Hearing deficits

55. Which of the following is not a sign or symptom caused by cubital tunnel syndrome?
A: Loss of lumbricals
B: Paresthesia in digit V.
C: Pain with elbow flexion
D: Abnormal Flexor carpi ulnaris strength

56. Which of the following medications is not considered a neuromuscular blocker?
A: Anectine
B: Pavulon
C: Pitressin
D: Mivacron

57. An occupational therapist is caring for a 10 year-old boy who has just been diagnosed with a congenital heart defect. Which of the following clinical signs does not indicate CHF?
A: Increased body weight
B: Elevated heart rate
C: Lower extremity edema
D: Compulsive behavior

58. An occupational therapist working in a pediatric clinic and observes the following situations. Which of the following may indicate a delayed child to the occupational therapist?

- 134 -

A: A 12-month old that does not "cruise".
B: A 8-month old that can sit upright unsupported.
C: A 6-month old that is rolling prone to supine.
D: A 3-month old that does not roll supine to prone.

59. An occupational therapist is reviewing a patient's current Lithium levels. Which of the following values is outside the therapeutic range?
A: 1.0 mEq/L
B: 1.1 mEq/L
C: 1.2 mEq/L
D: 1.3 mEq/L

60. Which of the following describes radial tunnel syndrome?
A: Compression of the Anterior Interosseous Nerve
B: Compression of the Posterior Interosseous Nerve
C: Crutch Palsy
D: Cubital Tunnel Syndrome

61. A patient has been ordered to get Klonapin for the first time. Which of the following side effects is not associated with Klonapin?
A: Drowsiness
B: Ataxia
C: Salivation elevated
D: Diplopia

62. A patient has been diagnosed with diabetes mellitus. Which of the following is not a clinical sign of diabetes mellitus?
A: Polyphagia
B: Polyuria
C: Metabolic acidosis
D: Lower extremity edema

63. A patient has fallen off a bicycle and fractured the distal radius with an avulsion of the ulna styloid. Which of the following terms would apply?
A: DeQuervain's Syndrome
B: Colles fracture
C: Gamekeeper's fracture
D: Mallet finger

64. Which of the following motions is identified with the corresponding action?
(Action- Turning palm of hand over to face in the anterior direction, dorsum of the hand is pointed downward toward the floor.)
A: Pronation
B: Supination
C: Abduction
D: Adduction

65. An occupational therapist is caring for a retired MD. The MD asks the question, "What type of cells secrete insulin?" The correct answer is:

A: alpha cells
B: beta cells
C: CD4 cells
D: helper cells

66. Which of the following is not considered one of the main mechanisms of Type II Diabetes treatment?
A: Medications
B: Nutrition
C: Increased activity
D: Continuous Insulin

67. An occupational therapist is caring for a retired MD. The MD asks the question, "What type of cells create exocrine secretions?" The correct answer is:
A: alpha cells
B: beta cells
C: acinar cells
D: plasma cells

68. An occupational therapist is caring for a patient who has experienced burns to the right upper extremity. According to the Rule of Nines which of the following percents most accurately describes the severity of the injury?
A: 36%
B: 27%
C: 18%
D: 9%

69. A patient has experienced a severe third degree burn to the trunk in the last 36 hours. Which phase of burn management is the patient in?
A: Shock phase
B: Emergent phase
C: Healing phase
D: Wound proliferation phase

70. An occupational therapist is reviewing a patient's medical record. The record indicates the patient has limited shoulder flexion on the left. Which plane of movement is limited?
A: Horizontal
B: Sagittal
C: Frontal
D: Vertical

71. A client is 72 hours post-op a TKR surgery. The occupational therapist notices that 270 cc's of sero-sanguinous accumulates in the surgical drains. What action should the occupational therapist take?
A: Notify the doctor
B: Empty the drain
C: Do nothing
D: Remove the drain

72. An occupational therapist is assigned to do home education teaching to a blind patient who is scheduled for discharge the following morning. What teaching strategy would best fit the situation?
A: Verbal teaching in short sessions throughout the day
B: Pre-operative booklet on the surgery in Braille
C: Provide a tape for the client
D: Have the blind patient's family member instruct the patient.

73. A violation of a patient's confidentiality occurs if two occupational therapists are discussing client information in which of the following scenarios?
A: With a occupational therapist treating the patient
B: With a social worker planning for discharge
C: With another occupational therapist on duty to plan for break time
D: In the hallway outside the patient's room.

74. If your patient is acutely psychotic, which of the following independent interventions would not be appropriate?
A: Conveying calmness with one on one interaction
B: Recognizing and dealing with your own feelings to prevent escalation of the patient's anxiety level
C: Encourage client participation in group therapy
D: Listen and identify causes of their behavior

75. An occupational therapist runs into the significant other of a patient with end stage AIDS crying during her smoke break. Which of the following is most appropriate action for the occupational therapist to take?
A: Allow her to grieve by herself.
B: Tell her go ahead and cry, after all your husband's pretty bad off.
C: Tell her you realize how upset she is, but you don't want to talk about it now.
D: Approach her, offering tissues and encourage her to verbalize her feelings.

Answer Key
1. (B) Teres Minor, Infraspinatus, Supraspinatus, and Subscapularis make up the Rotator Cuff.
2. (B) The patient experiencing neurovascular changes should have the highest priority. Pain following a TKR is normal, and breakdown over the heels is a gradual process. Moreover, a subacute ankle sprain is almost never a medical emergency.
3. (B) Gamekeeper's thumb identifies this condition.
4. (B) Pain may be indicating neurovascular complication.
5. (B) Stimulation in the form of pictures may decrease signs of confusion.
6. (D) Adolescents exhibiting signs of sexual development and interest are normal.
7. (A) Aides should be competent on transfers.
8. (D) All protective measures must be worn, it is not required to double glove.
9. (A) Total flexion minus total extension = TAM score.
10. (C) Both the family and the patient should have the need for restraints explained to them.
11. (B) The suicide plan may have been decided.
12. (A) Thrush may be occurring and the patient may need Nystatin.
13. (B) Check the intake and output prior to making any decisions about patient care.
14. (A) Negative culture results would indicate absence of infection.
15. (A) Purse lip breathing will help decrease the volume of air expelled by increased bronchial airways.
16. (B) The Mantoux is the most accurate test to determine the presence of TB.

17. (D) The MRI will require supine positioning.
18. (A) The frontal lobe is responsible for behavior and emotions.
19. (C) The patient's safety should have the highest priority.
20. (A) Seclusion is your best option in this scenario.
21. (A) CBAN, cold, burn, ache, numbness
22. (B) A ninhydrin test is used to check a patient's ability to sweat.
23. (D) The patient is in a state of denial.
24. (B) Fainting and hypotension can be caused by Tricyclics.
25. (B) Palpitations and muscle weakness are found with excessive levels of Digitalis.
26. (B) All of the clinical signs indicate a hyperglycemic condition.
27. (D) Anxiety is a clinical sign associated with respiratory acidosis.
28. (D) <200 T4 cells/deciliter
29. (C) Contacting the attending physician via the medical record is appropriate due to the possibility of melanoma.
30. (A) The patient is at high risk of developing increased intracranial pressure (ICP).
31. (B) The time slots and daily container would be the best recommendation in this case.
32. (C) Muscle weakness in the lower extremities is found in acute cases of Guillain-Barre' Syndrome.
33. (A) The shunt may be blocked and require immediate medical attention.
34. (A) LOC is the most critical indicator of impaired neurological capabilities.
35. (A) Patient safety should be the top concern about this patient.
36. (B) Unilateral pupil changes indicate changes in ICP.
37. (D) Left sided heart failure exhibits signs of pulmonary compromise (SOB).
38. (C) Some facilities require the physician to be notified about a patient's request and written permission from the husband is required for the wife to view the chart.
39. (D) Meal preparation is a multi-level problem solving situation.
40. (A) Hypotension may be result of over correction of a hypertensive condition.
41. (B) All of these criteria match up with a Swan Neck Deformity.
42. (C) Calcium is the most recognized osteoporosis treatment.
43. (D) Atropine encourages increased rate of conduction in the AV node.
44. (B) Lidocaine Hydrochloride can cause fatigue and confusion if an over dosage occurs.
45. (D) The spinner knob is your best recommendation given these parameters.
46. (A) Erythema with the skin intact can indicate a Stage I pressure ulcer.
47. (D) The moro reflex has all of the listed characteristics.
48. (B) The facial nerve (VII) is motor to the face and sensory to the anterior tongue.
49. (B) 60-115 mg/dl is standard range for serum glucose levels.
50. (C) Separation anxiety can easily occur after six months during hospitalization.
51. (D) Neural warmth will help to lower the baby's agitation level.
52. (D) An atlanto-axial dislocation may have occurred. Position the child in a neutral c-spine posture and then contact the doctor immediately.
53. (D) At one year this skill should be developed.
54. (A) Cognitive changes may include confusion and disorientation.
55. (A) FCU strength is fine in most cases.
56. (C) Pitressin is a hormone replacement medication.
57. (D) Compulsive behavior does not indicate CHF.
58. (A) At 12 months a child should at least be "cruising" (holding on to objects to walk). Cruising is considered pre-walking.
59. (D) 1.0-1.2 mEq/L is considered standard therapeutic range for patient care.
60. (B) Posterior Interosseous Nerve compression can cause RTS.
61. (D) A-C are associated side effects of Klonapin.

62. (D) A-C are associated with diabetes mellitus.

63. (B) These descriptions match up with a colles fracture.

64. (B) Supination- "Holding a bowl of soup in your hand."

65. (B) Beta cells secrete insulin.

66. (D) Insulin is not required in continuous treatment for every Type II diabetic.

67. (C) Acinar cells create exocrine secretions.

68. (D) Each arm is scored as 9% according to the Rule of Nines.

69. (A) The shock phase is considered the first 24-48 hours in wound management.

70. (B) Sagittal motion occurs in the midline plane of the body.

71. (A) The physician should be notified if excessive drainage is noted from the surgical site.

72. (A) Information is smaller amounts is easier to retain. Teaching the day before the discharge is best accomplished in a one on one format.

73. (D) Hallway discussions should not occur, because you do not who is listening, even though it may be a professional discussion.

74. (C) Acutely psychotic patients will disrupt group activities.

75. (D) Being left alone during the grief process, isolates individuals. These individuals need an outlet for their feelings and to talk to someone who is empathetic.

Secret Key #1 - Time is Your Greatest Enemy

Pace Yourself

Wear a watch. At the beginning of the test, check the time (or start a chronometer on your watch to count the minutes), and check the time after every few questions to make sure you are "on schedule."

If you are forced to speed up, do it efficiently. Usually one or more answer choices can be eliminated without too much difficulty. Above all, don't panic. Don't speed up and just begin guessing at random choices. By pacing yourself, and continually monitoring your progress against your watch, you will always know exactly how far ahead or behind you are with your available time. If you find that you are one minute behind on the test, don't skip one question without spending any time on it, just to catch back up. Take 15 fewer seconds on the next four questions, and after four questions you'll have caught back up. Once you catch back up, you can continue working each problem at your normal pace.

Furthermore, don't dwell on the problems that you were rushed on. If a problem was taking up too much time and you made a hurried guess, it must be difficult. The difficult questions are the ones you are most likely to miss anyway, so it isn't a big loss. It is better to end with more time than you need than to run out of time.

Lastly, sometimes it is beneficial to slow down if you are constantly getting ahead of time. You are always more likely to catch a careless mistake by working more slowly than quickly, and among very high-scoring test takers (those who are likely to have lots of time left over), careless errors affect the score more than mastery of material.

Secret Key #2 - Guessing is not Guesswork

You probably know that guessing is a good idea - unlike other standardized tests, there is no penalty for getting a wrong answer. Even if you have no idea about a question, you still have a 20-25% chance of getting it right.

Most test takers do not understand the impact that proper guessing can have on their score. Unless you score extremely high, guessing will significantly contribute to your final score.

Monkeys Take the Test

What most test takers don't realize is that to insure that 20-25% chance, you have to guess randomly. If you put 20 monkeys in a room to take this test, assuming they answered once per question and behaved themselves, on average they would get 20-25% of the questions correct. Put 20 test takers in the room, and the average will be much lower among guessed questions. Why?

1. The test writers intentionally writes deceptive answer choices that "look" right. A test taker has no idea about a question, so picks the "best looking" answer, which is often wrong. The monkey has no idea what looks good and what doesn't, so will consistently be lucky about 20-25% of the time.
2. Test takers will eliminate answer choices from the guessing pool based on a hunch or intuition. Simple but correct answers often get excluded, leaving a 0% chance of being correct. The monkey has no clue, and often gets lucky with the best choice.

This is why the process of elimination endorsed by most test courses is flawed and detrimental to your performance- test takers don't guess, they make an ignorant stab in the dark that is usually worse than random.

$5 Challenge

Let me introduce one of the most valuable ideas of this course- the $5 challenge:

You only mark your "best guess" if you are willing to bet $5 on it.
You only eliminate choices from guessing if you are willing to bet $5 on it.

Why $5? Five dollars is an amount of money that is small yet not insignificant, and can really add up fast (20 questions could cost you $100). Likewise, each answer choice on one question of the test will have a small impact on your overall score, but it can really add up to a lot of points in the end.

The process of elimination IS valuable. The following shows your chance of guessing it right:

If you eliminate wrong answer choices until only this many answer choices remain:	1	2	3
Chance of getting it correct:	100%	50%	33%

However, if you accidentally eliminate the right answer or go on a hunch for an incorrect answer, your chances drop dramatically: to 0%. By guessing among all the answer choices, you are GUARANTEED to have a shot at the right answer.

That's why the $5 test is so valuable- if you give up the advantage and safety of a pure guess, it had better be worth the risk.

What we still haven't covered is how to be sure that whatever guess you make is truly random. Here's the easiest way:

Always pick the first answer choice among those remaining.

Such a technique means that you have decided, **before you see a single test question**, exactly how you are going to guess- and since the order of choices tells you nothing about which one is correct, this guessing technique is perfectly random.

This section is not meant to scare you away from making educated guesses or eliminating choices- you just need to define when a choice is worth eliminating. The $5 test, along with a pre-defined random guessing strategy, is the best way to make sure you reap all of the benefits of guessing.

Secret Key #3 - Practice Smarter, Not Harder

Many test takers delay the test preparation process because they dread the awful amounts of practice time they think necessary to succeed on the test. We have refined an effective method that will take you only a fraction of the time.

There are a number of "obstacles" in your way to succeed. Among these are answering questions, finishing in time, and mastering test-taking strategies. All must be executed on the day of the test at peak performance, or your score will suffer. The test is a mental marathon that has a large impact on your future.

Just like a marathon runner, it is important to work your way up to the full challenge. So first you just worry about questions, and then time, and finally strategy:

Success Strategy

1. Find a good source for practice tests.
2. If you are willing to make a larger time investment, consider using more than one study guide-often the different approaches of multiple authors will help you "get" difficult concepts.
3. Take a practice test with no time constraints, with all study helps "open book." Take your time with questions and focus on applying strategies.
4. Take a practice test with time constraints, with all guides "open book."
5. Take a final practice test with no open material and time limits

If you have time to take more practice tests, just repeat step 5. By gradually exposing yourself to the full rigors of the test environment, you will condition your mind to the stress of test day and maximize your success.

Secret Key #4 - Prepare, Don't Procrastinate

Let me state an obvious fact: if you take the test three times, you will get three different scores. This is due to the way you feel on test day, the level of preparedness you have, and, despite the test writers' claims to the contrary, some tests WILL be easier for you than others.

Since your future depends so much on your score, you should maximize your chances of success. In order to maximize the likelihood of success, you've got to prepare in advance. This means taking practice tests and spending time learning the information and test taking strategies you will need to succeed.

Never take the test as a "practice" test, expecting that you can just take it again if you need to. Feel free to take sample tests on your own, but when you go to take the official test, be prepared, be focused, and do your best the first time!

Secret Key #5 - Test Yourself

Everyone knows that time is money. There is no need to spend too much of your time or too little of your time preparing for the test. You should only spend as much of your precious time preparing as is necessary for you to get the score you need.

Once you have taken a practice test under real conditions of time constraints, then you will know if you are ready for the test or not.

If you have scored extremely high the first time that you take the practice test, then there is not much point in spending countless hours studying. You are already there.

Benchmark your abilities by retaking practice tests and seeing how much you have improved. Once you score high enough to guarantee success, then you are ready.

If you have scored well below where you need, then knuckle down and begin studying in earnest. Check your improvement regularly through the use of practice tests under real conditions. Above all, don't worry, panic, or give up. The key is perseverance!

Then, when you go to take the test, remain confident and remember how well you did on the practice tests. If you can score high enough on a practice test, then you can do the same on the real thing.

General Strategies

The most important thing you can do is to ignore your fears and jump into the test immediately- do not be overwhelmed by any strange-sounding terms. You have to jump into the test like jumping into a pool- all at once is the easiest way.

Make Predictions

As you read and understand the question, try to guess what the answer will be. Remember that several of the answer choices are wrong, and once you begin reading them, your mind will immediately become cluttered with answer choices designed to throw you off. Your mind is typically the most focused immediately after you have read the question and digested its contents. If you can, try to predict what the correct answer will be. You may be surprised at what you can predict.

Quickly scan the choices and see if your prediction is in the listed answer choices. If it is, then you can be quite confident that you have the right answer. It still won't hurt to check the other answer choices, but most of the time, you've got it!

Answer the Question

It may seem obvious to only pick answer choices that answer the question, but the test writers can create some excellent answer choices that are wrong. Don't pick an answer just because it sounds right, or you believe it to be true. It MUST answer the question. Once you've made your selection, always go back and check it against the question and make sure that you didn't misread the question, and the answer choice does answer the question posed.

Benchmark

After you read the first answer choice, decide if you think it sounds correct or not. If it doesn't, move on to the next answer choice. If it does, mentally mark that answer choice. This doesn't mean that you've definitely selected it as your answer choice, it just means that it's the best you've seen thus far. Go ahead and read the next choice. If the next choice is worse than the one you've already selected, keep going to the next answer choice. If the next choice is better than the choice you've already selected, mentally mark the new answer choice as your best guess.

The first answer choice that you select becomes your standard. Every other answer choice must be benchmarked against that standard. That choice is correct until proven otherwise by another answer choice beating it out. Once you've decided that no other answer choice seems as good, do one final check to ensure that your answer choice answers the question posed.

Valid Information

Don't discount any of the information provided in the question. Every piece of information may be necessary to determine the correct answer. None of the information in the question is there to throw you off (while the answer choices will certainly have information to throw you off). If two seemingly unrelated topics are discussed, don't ignore either. You can be confident there is a relationship, or it wouldn't be included in the question, and you are probably going to have to determine what is that relationship to find the answer.

Avoid "Fact Traps"

Don't get distracted by a choice that is factually true. Your search is for the answer that answers the question. Stay focused and don't fall for an answer that is true but incorrect. Always go back to the question and make sure you're choosing an answer that actually answers the question and is not just a true statement. An answer can be factually correct, but it MUST answer the question asked. Additionally, two answers can both be seemingly correct, so be sure to read all of the answer choices, and make sure that you get the one that BEST answers the question.

Milk the Question

Some of the questions may throw you completely off. They might deal with a subject you have not been exposed to, or one that you haven't reviewed in years. While your lack of knowledge about the subject will be a hindrance, the question itself can give you many clues that will help you find the correct answer. Read the question carefully and look for clues. Watch particularly for adjectives and nouns describing difficult terms or words that you don't recognize. Regardless of if you completely understand a word or not, replacing it with a synonym either provided or one you more familiar with may help you to understand what the questions are asking. Rather than wracking your mind about specific detailed information concerning a difficult term or word, try to use mental substitutes that are easier to understand.

The Trap of Familiarity

Don't just choose a word because you recognize it. On difficult questions, you may not recognize a number of words in the answer choices. The test writers don't put "make-believe" words on the test; so don't think that just because you only recognize all the words in one answer choice means that answer choice must be correct. If you only recognize words in one answer choice, then focus on that one. Is it correct? Try your best to determine if it is correct. If it is, that is great, but if it doesn't, eliminate it. Each word and answer choice you eliminate increases your chances of getting the question correct, even if you then have to guess among the unfamiliar choices.

Eliminate Answers

Eliminate choices as soon as you realize they are wrong. But be careful! Make sure you consider all of the possible answer choices. Just because one appears right, doesn't mean that the next one won't be even better! The test writers will usually put more than one good answer choice for every question, so read all of them. Don't worry if you are stuck between two that seem right. By getting down to just two remaining possible choices, your odds are now 50/50. Rather than wasting too much time, play the odds. You are guessing, but guessing wisely, because you've been able to knock out some of the answer choices that you know are wrong. If you are eliminating choices and realize that the last answer choice you are left with is also obviously wrong, don't panic. Start over and consider each choice again. There may easily be something that you missed the first time and will realize on the second pass.

Tough Questions

If you are stumped on a problem or it appears too hard or too difficult, don't waste time. Move on! Remember though, if you can quickly check for obviously incorrect answer choices, your chances of guessing correctly are greatly improved. Before you completely give up, at least try to knock out a couple of possible answers. Eliminate what you can and then guess at the remaining answer choices before moving on.

Brainstorm

If you get stuck on a difficult question, spend a few seconds quickly brainstorming. Run through the complete list of possible answer choices. Look at each choice and ask yourself, "Could this answer the question satisfactorily?" Go through each answer choice and consider it independently of the other. By systematically going through all possibilities, you may find something that you would otherwise overlook. Remember that when you get stuck, it's important to try to keep moving.

Read Carefully
Understand the problem. Read the question and answer choices carefully. Don't miss the question because you misread the terms. You have plenty of time to read each question thoroughly and make sure you understand what is being asked. Yet a happy medium must be attained, so don't waste too much time. You must read carefully, but efficiently.

Face Value
When in doubt, use common sense. Always accept the situation in the problem at face value. Don't read too much into it. These problems will not require you to make huge leaps of logic. The test writers aren't trying to throw you off with a cheap trick. If you have to go beyond creativity and make a leap of logic in order to have an answer choice answer the question, then you should look at the other answer choices. Don't overcomplicate the problem by creating theoretical relationships or explanations that will warp time or space. These are normal problems rooted in reality. It's just that the applicable relationship or explanation may not be readily apparent and you have to figure things out. Use your common sense to interpret anything that isn't clear.

Prefixes
If you're having trouble with a word in the question or answer choices, try dissecting it. Take advantage of every clue that the word might include. Prefixes and suffixes can be a huge help. Usually they allow you to determine a basic meaning. Pre- means before, post- means after, pro - is positive, de- is negative. From these prefixes and suffixes, you can get an idea of the general meaning of the word and try to put it into context. Beware though of any traps. Just because con is the opposite of pro, doesn't necessarily mean congress is the opposite of progress!

Hedge Phrases
Watch out for critical "hedge" phrases, such as likely, may, can, will often, sometimes, often, almost, mostly, usually, generally, rarely, sometimes. Question writers insert these hedge phrases to cover every possibility. Often an answer choice will be wrong simply because it leaves no room for exception. Avoid answer choices that have definitive words like "exactly," and "always".

Switchback Words
Stay alert for "switchbacks". These are the words and phrases frequently used to alert you to shifts in thought. The most common switchback word is "but". Others include although, however, nevertheless, on the other hand, even though, while, in spite of, despite, regardless of.

New Information
Correct answer choices will rarely have completely new information included. Answer choices typically are straightforward reflections of the material asked about and will directly relate to the question. If a new piece of information is included in an answer choice that doesn't even seem to relate to the topic being asked about, then that answer choice is likely incorrect. All of the information needed to answer the question is usually provided for you, and so you should not have to make guesses that are unsupported or choose answer choices that require unknown information that cannot be reasoned on its own.

Time Management
On technical questions, don't get lost on the technical terms. Don't spend too much time on any one question. If you don't know what a term means, then since you don't have a dictionary, odds are you

aren't going to get much further. You should immediately recognize terms as whether or not you know them. If you don't, work with the other clues that you have, the other answer choices and terms provided, but don't waste too much time trying to figure out a difficult term.

Contextual Clues

Look for contextual clues. An answer can be right but not correct. The contextual clues will help you find the answer that is most right and is correct. Understand the context in which a phrase or statement is made. This will help you make important distinctions.

Don't Panic

Panicking will not answer any questions for you. Therefore, it isn't helpful. When you first see the question, if your mind goes blank, take a deep breath. Force yourself to mechanically go through the steps of solving the problem and using the strategies you've learned.

Pace Yourself

Don't get clock fever. It's easy to be overwhelmed when you're looking at a page full of questions, your mind is full of random thoughts and feeling confused, and the clock is ticking down faster than you would like. Calm down and maintain the pace that you have set for yourself. As long as you are on track by monitoring your pace, you are guaranteed to have enough time for yourself. When you get to the last few minutes of the test, it may seem like you won't have enough time left, but if you only have as many questions as you should have left at that point, then you're right on track!

Answer Selection

The best way to pick an answer choice is to eliminate all of those that are wrong, until only one is left and confirm that is the correct answer. Sometimes though, an answer choice may immediately look right. Be careful! Take a second to make sure that the other choices are not equally obvious. Don't make a hasty mistake. There are only two times that you should stop before checking other answers. First is when you are positive that the answer choice you have selected is correct. Second is when time is almost out and you have to make a quick guess!

Check Your Work

Since you will probably not know every term listed and the answer to every question, it is important that you get credit for the ones that you do know. Don't miss any questions through careless mistakes. If at all possible, try to take a second to look back over your answer selection and make sure you've selected the correct answer choice and haven't made a costly careless mistake (such as marking an answer choice that you didn't mean to mark). This quick double check should more than pay for itself in caught mistakes for the time it costs.

Beware of Directly Quoted Answers

Sometimes an answer choice will repeat word for word a portion of the question or reference section. However, beware of such exact duplication – it may be a trap! More than likely, the correct choice will paraphrase or summarize a point, rather than being exactly the same wording.

Slang

Scientific sounding answers are better than slang ones. An answer choice that begins "To compare the outcomes…" is much more likely to be correct than one that begins "Because some people insisted…"

Extreme Statements

Avoid wild answers that throw out highly controversial ideas that are proclaimed as established fact. An answer choice that states the "process should be used in certain situations, if…" is much more likely to be correct than one that states the "process should be discontinued completely." The first is a calm rational statement and doesn't even make a definitive, uncompromising stance, using a hedge word "if" to provide wiggle room, whereas the second choice is a radical idea and far more extreme.

Answer Choice Families
When you have two or more answer choices that are direct opposites or parallels, one of them is usually the correct answer. For instance, if one answer choice states "x increases" and another answer choice states "x decreases" or "y increases," then those two or three answer choices are very similar in construction and fall into the same family of answer choices. A family of answer choices is when two or three answer choices are very similar in construction, and yet often have a directly opposite meaning. Usually the correct answer choice will be in that family of answer choices. The "odd man out" or answer choice that doesn't seem to fit the parallel construction of the other answer choices is more likely to be incorrect.

	Tubercle, Below and Medial to the Radial Groove		
Anconeus	Posterior, Lateral Humeral Condyle	Upper Posterior Ulna	Radial
Brachioradialis	Lateral Supracondylar Ridge of Humerus	Radial Styloid Process	Radial
Pronator Teres	Medial Epicondyle and Supracondylar Ridge	½ Way Down on Lateral Radius	Median
Pronator Quadratus	Distal-Medial Ulna	Distal-Lateral Radius	Anterior Interosseous

Review of the Forearm

Muscle	Origin	Insertion	Nerve
Brachioradialis	Lateral Supracondylar Ridge of Humerus	Radial Styloid Process	Radial
Pronator Teres	Medial Epicondyle and Supracondylar Ridge	½ Way Down on Lateral Radius	Median
Pronator Quadratus	Distal-Medial Ulna	Distal-Lateral Radius	Anterior Interosseous
Supinator	Lateral Epicondyle of Humerus	Upper ½ Lateral, Posterior Radius	Posterior Inter-Deep Radial
Flexor Carpi Radialis	Medial Epicondyle of Humerus	2nd and 3rd Metacarpal	Median
Flexor Carpi Ulnaris	Medial Epicondyle of Humerus	Pisiform, Hamate, 5th Metacarpal	Ulnar
Palmaris Longus	Medial Epicondyle of the Humerus	Palmar Aponeurosis and Flexor Retinaculum	Median
Flexor Digitorum Suerficialis	Medial Epicondyle, Radius, Ulna	Medial 4 Digits	Median
Flexor Digitorum Profundus	Ulna, Interosseous Membrane	Medial 4 Digits (distal part)	Median (lateral 2 digits), Ulnar (median 2 digits)
Flexor Pollicis Longus	Radius	Distal Phalanx (thumb)	Anterior Inter-Deep Median
Extensor Carpi Radialis Longus	Lateral Condyle and Supracondylar Ridge	2nd Metacarpal	Radial
Extensor Carpi Radialis Brevis	Lateral Epicondyle of Humerus	3rd Metacarpal	Posterior Inter-Deep Radial
Extensor Carpi Ulnaris	Lateral Epicondyle of Humerus	5th Metacarpal	Posterior Inter-Deep Radial
Extensor Digitorum	Lateral Epicondyle of	Extension Expansion	Posterior Inter-Deep

	Humerus	Hood of Medial 4 Digits	Radial
Extensor Digiti Minimi	Lateral Epicondyle of Humerus	Extension Expansion Hood of (little finger)	Posterior Inter-Deep Radial
Abductor Pollicis Longus	Posterior Radius and Ulna	Radial Side of 1st Metacarpal	Posterior Inter-Deep Radial
Extensor Indicis	Ulna and Interosseous Membrane	Extension Expansion Hood (index finger)	Posterior Inter-Deep Radial
Extensor Pollicis Longus	Ulna and Interosseous Membrane	Distal Phalanx (thumb)	Posterior Inter-Deep Radial
Extensor Pollicis Brevis	Radius	Proximal Phalanx (thumb)	Posterior Inter-Deep Radial

Review of the Hand

Muscle	Origin	Insertion	Nerve
Adductor Policis	Capitate and Base of Adjacent Metacarpals	Proximal Phalanx (thumb)	Deep Branch of Ulnar
Lumbricals	Tendons of Flexor Digitorum Profundas	Extension Expansion Hood of Medial 4 Digits	Deep Branch Ulnar (medial 2 Ls), Median (lateral 2 Ls)
Dorsal Interosseous Muscles (4)	Sides of Metacarpals	Extension Expansion Hood of Digits 2-4	Deep Branch Ulnar
Palmar Interosseous (3)	Sides of Metacarpals	Extension Expansion Hood, Digits 2,4,5	Deep Branch Ulnar
Palmaris Brevis	Anterior Flexor Retinaculum and Palmar Aponeurosis	Skin-Ulnar Border of Hand	Superficial Ulnar
Abductor Pollicis Brevis	Flexor Retinaculum, Trapezium	Lateral Proximal Phalanx (thumb)	Median (thenar branch)
Flexor Pollicis Brevis	Flexor Retinaculum, Trapezium	Lateral Proximal Phalanx (thumb)	Median (thenar branch)
Opponens Pollicis	Flexor Retinaculum, Trapezium	Radial Border (1st Metacarpal)	Median (thenar branch)
Abductor Digiti Minimi	Flexor Retinaculum, Pisiform	Proximal Phalanx (little finger)	Deep Branch Ulnar
Flexor Digiti Minimi	Flexor Retinaculum, Hamate	Proximal Phalanx (little finger)	Deep Branch Ulnar
Opponens Digiti Minimi	Flexor Retinaculum, Hamate	Ulnar Medial Border (5th Metacarpal)	Deep Branch Ulnar

Review of the Thigh

Muscle	Origin	Insertion	Nerve

- 152 -

Psoas Major	Bodies and Discs of T12-L5	Lesser Trochanter	L2,3
Psoas Minor	Bodies and Discs of T12 and L1	Pectineal Line of Superior Pubic Bone	L2,3
Iliacus	Upper 2/3 Iliac Fossa	Lesser Trochanter	Femoral L2-4
Pectinius	Pubic Ramus	Spiral Line	Femoral
Iliposoas	Joining of Psoas Major and Iliacus	Lesser Trochanter	L2-4
Piriformis	Anterior Surface of the Sacrum	Greater Trochanter	S1, S2
Obturator Internus	Inner Surface of the Obturator Membrane	Greater Trochanter	Sacral Plexus
Obturator Externus	Outer Surface of the Obturator Membrane	Greater Trochanter	Obturator
Gemellus Superior	Ischial Spine	Greater Trochanter	Sacral Plexus
Gemellus Inferior	Ischial Tuberosity	Greater Trochanter	Sacral Plexus
Quadratus Femoris	Ischial Tuberosity	Quadrate Tubercle of the Femur	Sacral Plexus
Gluteus Maximus	Outer Surface of Ilium, Sacrum and Coccyx	Iliotibial Tract, Gluteal Tubercle of the Femur	Inferior Gluteal
Gluteus Minimus	Outer Surface of the Ilium	Greater Trochanter	Superior Gluteal
Gluteus Medius	Outer Surface of the Ilium	Greater Trochanter	Superior Gluteal
Satorius	Anterior Superior Iliac Spine	Upper Medial Tibia	Femoral
Quadriceps Femoris	Anterior Inferior Iliac Spine, Femur-Lateral and Medial	Tibial Tuberosity	Femoral
Gracilis	Pubic Bone	Upper Medial Tibia	Obturator (anterior branch)
Abductor Longus	Pubic Bone	Linea Aspera	Obturator (anterior branch)
Abductor Brevis	Pubic Bone	Linea Aspera	Obturator (anterior branch)
Abductor Magnus	Pubic Bone	Entire Linea Aspera	Sciatic, Obturator
Tensor Faciae Latae	Iliac Crest	Iliotibial Band	Superior Gluteal
Biceps Femoris	Ischial Tuberosity, Linea Aspera	Head of Fibula, Lateral Condyle of Tibia	Sciatic-Tibial portion and Common Peroneal Portion
Semimembranosus	Ischial Tuberosity	Upper Medial Tibia	Sciatic-Tibial Portion
Semitendinosus	Ischial Tuberosity	Upper Medial Tibia	Sciatic-Tibial Portion

- 153 -

Review of the Calf and Foot

Muscle	Origin	Insertion	Nerve
Tibialis Anterior	Upper 2/3 Lateral Tibia and Interosseous Membrane	1st Cuneiform and Base of 1st Metatarsal	Deep Peroneal
Extensor Digitorum Longus	Upper 2/3 Fibula and Interosseous Membrane	4 Tendons-Distal Middle Phalanges	Deep Peroneal
Extensor Hallucis Longus	Middle 1/3 of Anterior Fibula	Base of Distal Phalanx of Big Toe	Deep Peroneal
Peroneus Tertius	Distal Fibula	Base of 5th Metatarsal	Deep Peroneal
Extensor Hallucis Brevis	Dorsal Calcaneus	Extensor Digitorum Longus Tendons	Deep Peroneal
Peroneus Longus	Upper 2/3 Lateral Fibula	1st Metatarsal and 1st Cuneiform	Superficial Peroneal
Peroneus Brevis	Lateral Distal Fibula	5th Metatarsal Tuberosity	Superficial Peroneal
Soleus	Upper Shaft of Fibula	Calcaneus via Achilles Tendon	Tibial
Flexor Digitorum Longus	Middle 1/3 of Posterior Tibia	Base of Distal Phalanx of Lateral 4 Toes	Tibial
Flexor Hallucis Longus	Middle and Lower 1/3 of Posterior Tibia	Distal Phalanx of Big Toe	Tibial
Tibialis Posterior	Posterior Upper Tibia, Fibula	Navicular Bone and 1st Cuneiform	Tibial
Popliteus	Upper Posterior Tibia	Lateral Condyle of Femur	Tibial
Flexor Digitorum Brevis	Calcaneus	Middle Phalanges of Lateral 4 Toes	Medial Plantar
Abductor Hallucis	Calcaneus	Medial Proximal Phalanx of Big Toe	Medial Plantar
Abductor Digiti Brevis	Calcaneus	Lateral Proximal Phalanx of Big Toe	Lateral Plantar
Quadratus Plantae	Lateral and Medial Side of the Calcaneus	Tendons of Flexor Digitorum Longus	Lateral Plantar
Lumbricals	Tendons of Flexor Digitorum Longus	Extensor Tendons of Toes	Medial Plantar/Lateral Plantar
Flexor Hallucis Brevis	Cuboid Bone	Splits on Base of Proximal Phalanx of Big Toe	Medial Plantar
Flexor Digiti Minimi Brevis	Base of 5th Metatarsal	Base of Proximal Phalanx of Little Toe	Lateral Plantar

Abductor Hallucis	Metatarsals 2-4	Base of Proximal Phalanx of Big Toe	Lateral Plantar
Interossei	Sides of Metatarsal Bones	Base of 1st Phalanx and Extensor Tendons	Lateral Plantar

Special Report: Quick Reference Lesion Review

Occipital Lobe	Homonymous hemianopsia, partial seizures with limited visual phenomena
Thalamus	Contralateral thalamus pain, contralateral hemisensory loss
Pineal gland	Early hydrocephalus, papillary abnormalities, Parinaud's syndrome
Internal capsule	Hemisensory loss, homonymous hemianopsia, contralateral hemiplegia
Basal ganglia	Contralateral dystonia, Contralateral choreoathetosis
Pons	Diplopia, internal strabismus, VI and VII involvement, contralateral hemisensory and hemiparesis loss, issilateral cerebellar ataxia
Broca's area	Motor dysphasia
Precentral gyrus	Jacksonian seizures, generalized seizures, hemiparesis
Superficial parietal lobe	Receptive dysphasia
Cerebellar hemisphere	Ipsilateral cerebellar ataxia with hypotonia, dysmetria, intention tremor, nystagmus to side of lesion
Midbrain	Loss of upward gaze, III involvement, ipsilateral cerebellar signs, diplopia
Angular gyrus	Finger agnosia, allochiria, agraphia, acalculia
Temporal lobe	Contralateral homonymous upper quadrantanopsia, partial complex seizures
Paracentral lobe	Urgency of micturition, incontinence, progressive spastic paraparesis
Third Ventricle	Hydrocephalus
Fourth Ventricle	Hydrocephalus, progressive spastic hemiparesis
Optic Chiasm	Bitemporal hemianopsia, optic atrophy
Uncus	Partial complex seizures
Superior temporal gyrus	Receptive dysphasia
Prefrontal area	Apathy, poor attention span, loss of judgement, release phenomena, distractible
Orbital surface frontal lobe	Paroxysmal atrial tachycardia
Hypothalmus	Amenorrhea, cachexia, hypopituitarism, hypothyrodism, impotence, diencephalic autonomic seizures

Special Report: Normal Lab Values

Hematologic	
Bleeding time (template)	Less than 10 minutes
Erythrocyte count	4.2-5.9 million/cu mm
Erythrocyte sedimentation rate (Westergren)	Male: 0-15 mm/hr; female: 0-20 mm/hr
Hematocrit, blood	Male: 42-50%; female: 40-48%
Hemoglobin, blood	Male: 13-16 g/dL; female: 12-15 g/dL
Leukocyte count and differential	Leukocyte count: 4000-11,000/cu mm; 50-70% segmented neutrophils; 0-5% band forms, 0-3% eosinophils, 0-1% basophils, 30-45% lymphocytes, 0-6% monocytes
Mean corpuscular volume	86-98 fL
Prothrombin time, plasma	11-13 seconds
Partial thromboplastin time (activated)	30-40 seconds
Platelet count	150,000-300,000/cu mm
Reticulocyte count	0.5-1.5% of red cells
Whole blood, Plasma, serum chemistries	
Amylase, serum	25-125 U/L
Arterial studies, blood (patient breathing room air)	
PO2	75-100 mm Hg
PCO2	38-42 mm Hg
Bicarbonate	23-26 mEq/L
pH	7.38-7.44
Oxygen saturation	95% or greater
Bicarbonate, serum	23-28 mEq/L
Bilirubin, serum:	
Total	0.3-1.0 mg/dL
Direct	0.1-0.3 mg/dL
Comprehensive metabolic panel:	
Bilirubin, serum (total)	0.3-1.0 mg/dL
Calcium, serum	Male: 9.0-10.5 mg/dL; female: 8.5-10.2 mg/dL
Cholesterol, serum (total)	Desirable: less than 200 mg/dL Borderline-high: 200-239 mg/dL (may be high in the presence of coronary artery disease or other risk factors) High: greater than 239 mg/dL
Creatinine, serum	0.7-1.5 mg/dL

Glucose, plasma	Normal (fasting): 70-115 mg/dL
	Borderline: 115-140 mg/dL
	Abnormal: greater than 140 mg/dL
Phosphorus, serum	3.0-4.5 mg/dL
Proteins, serum:	
Pre-Albumin	.2 - 0.4 g/dL
Albumin	3.5-5.5 g/dL
Urea nitrogen, blood (BUN)	8-20 mg/dL
Uric acid, serum	3.0-7.0 mg/dL
Calcium, serum	Male: 9.0-10.5 mg/dL: female: 8.5-10.2 mg/dL
Chloride, serum	98-106 mEq/L
Cholesterol, serum:	Desirable: less than 200 mg/dL
Total	Borderline-high: 200-239 mg/dL (may be high in the presence of coronary artery disease or other risk factors)
	High: greater than 239 mg/dL
High-density lipoprotein	Low: less than 40 mg/dL
Low-density lipoprotein	Optimal: less than 100 mg/dL
	Near-optimal: 100-129 mg/dL
	Borderline-high: 130-159 mg/dL (may be high in the presence of coronary artery disease or other risk factors)
	High: 160-189 mg/dL
	Very high: 190 mg/dL and above
Creatinine, serum	0.7-1.5 mg/dL
Electrolytes, serum:	
Sodium	136-145 mEq/L
Potassium	3.5-5.0 mEq/L
Chloride	98-106 mEq/L
Bicarbonate	23-28 mEq/L
Follicle-stimulating hormone, serum	Adult male: 2-18 mLU/mL
	Female: 5-20 mLU/mL (follicular or luteal)
	30-50 mLU/mL (mid-cycle peak)
	greater than 50 mLU/mL (postmenopausal)
Glucose, plasma	Normal (fasting): 70-115 mg/dL
	Borderline: 115-140 mg/dL
	Abnormal: greater than 140 mg/dL
Lactate dehydrogenase, serum	140-280 U/L
Osmolality, serum	280-300 mOsm/kg H2O
Oxygen saturation, arterial blood	95% or greater
Phosphatase (alkaline), serum	30-120 U/L
Phosphorus, serum	3.0-4.5 mg/dL

Potassium, serum   3.5-5.0 mEq/L

Proteins, serum:

Sodium, serum   136-145 mEq/L

Triglycerides, serum (fasting)   Normal: less than 250 mg/dL
                                                Borderline: 250-500 mg/dL
                                                Abnormal: greater than 500 mg/dL

Urea nitrogen, blood   8-20 mg/dL

Uric acid. Serum   3.0-7.0 mg/dL

Special Report: Myotome and Dermatome Screening Reference

Myotome Screening Cervical	(ASIA) Scale
C1-2	Neck flexion/extension
C3	Lateral neck flexion
C4	Shoulder Shrug
C5	Elbow flexors
C6	Wrist extensors
C7	Triceps
T1	Finger flexion

Dermatome Screening Cervical	(ASIA) Scale
C4	Deltoid Region
C5	Lateral Arm
C6	Lateral Forearm
C7	Middle Finger
C8	Digits 4/5
T1	Medial forearm
T2	Axilla Region

Myotome Screening Lumbar	(ASIA) Scale
L2	Hip flexors
L3	Knee Extension
L4	Ankle Dorsiflexion
L5	Great Toe Extension
S1	Plantar flexion

Dermatome Screening Lumbar	(ASIA) Scale
L1	Groin (Lateral>Medial)
L2	Upper Anterior Thigh
L3	Lower Anterior Thigh
L4	Knee/Medial leg
L5	Lateral leg/web space
S1	Lateral ankle/foot

Special Report: High Frequency Terms

The following terms were compiled as high frequency NBCOT test terms. I recommend printing out this list and identifying the terms you are unfamiliar with. Then, use a medical dictionary or the internet to look up the terms you have questions about. Take one section per day if you have the time to maximize recall.

A

Acquired immunodeficiency syndrome
Aneurysm
Angina pectoris
Angiogenesis
Anklyosing spondylitis
Anterior Interosseous Syndrome
Anxiety
Appendicitis
Arterial disease
Arteriosclerosis
Arthralgia
Arthritis
Atypical angina
AZT

B

Back pain
Blood cultures
Boutonniere Deformity
Bradycardia
Braxton-Hicks contractions
Bronchiectasis
Bulimia

C

CAD
Cancer
Cardiac disease
Carpal tunnel syndrome
Chest pain
Chest x-ray
Cirrhosis
Claw fingers
COLD
Colles Fracture
Cubital tunnel Syndrome
Corticosteroids

D

Degenerative heart disease
DeQuervain's syndrome

Diabetes insipidus
Diabetes mellitus
Diabetic nephropathy
Dialysis
Diaphoresis
Down's syndrome
Dupuytran's contracture
DVT
Dyspnea

E
Ectopic pregnancy
Electrocardiogram (ECG)
Embolism
Emphysema
Endocrine system
Epinephrine
Esophagitis

F
Fatigue
Fibrillation
Fibromyalgia syndrome

G

Gamekeeper's thumb
Gangrene
Ganglion
Glucagon
Glucose tolerance test
Guillai-Barre' syndrome

H
Heart failure
Heart rate
Hemophilia
Hemorrhage
Heparin
Herpes zoster
Hiatal hernia
HIV
Hyponatremia
Hypothyroidism
Hypoxia
Hysterectomy

I

Induration
Inflammatory bowel disease
Inhibitors
Ischemic Heart Disease

J

Jaundice
Joint pain
Joint sepsis
Jevenile rheumatoid arthritis

K

Kidney failure
Kidney stones

L

Labile hypertension
Lactation
Low back pain
Lymphocyctes

M

Macrophages
Mallet finger
Menarche
Ménière's disease
Metabolism
Multiple sclerosis
Myalgias

N

Neck pain
Neomycin
Night sweats
Nitrates
Nitroglycerin
Nocturnal angina
Norepinephrine
Nystagmus

O

Orthostatic hypotension
Osteoarthritis

Osteoporosis

P
Pain–joint
Palmar erythema
Palpitations
Pancreatitis
Parathyroid hormone
Paresthesia
Parkinson's disease
Pelvic inflammatory disease (PID)
Pericarditis
Pregnancy
Psychological support
Pulmonary edema

Q
Quadriceps

R
RA- Rheumatoid arthritis
Referred pain
Reflex sympathetic dystrophy
Renal failure
Respiration
Rheumatic fever
Right ventricular failure

S
Scaphoid Fx.
Sciatica
Scleroderma
Shoulder pain
Sickle cell anemia
Sinus bradycardia
Sinus tachycardia
Smoking
Swan neck deformity
Systolic rate

T
Tendinitis
Thyroid gland
Tissue necrosis
Trauma
Tuberculosis

U
Ulceration
Umbilical pain
Ureter obstruction
Urinary tract infection

V

Ventricular failure
Vertigo
Vital signs
Vomiting

W
Weight gain

CPR Review/Cheat Sheet

Topic	New Guidelines
Conscious Choking	5 back blows, then 5 abdominal thrusts- adult/child
Unconscious Choking	5 chest compressions, look, 2 breaths-adult/child/infant
Rescue Breaths	Normal Breath given over 1 second until chest rises
Chest Compressions to Ventilation Ratios (Single Rescuer)	30:2 – Adult/Child/Infant
Chest Compressions to Ventilation Ratios (Two Rescuer)	30:2 – Adult 15:2 – Child/Infant
Chest Compression rate	About 100/minute – Adult/Child/Infant
Chest Compression Land marking Method	Simplified approach – center of the chest – Adult/Child 2 or 3 fingers, just below the nipple line at the center of the chest - Infant
AED	1 shock, then 2 minutes (or 5 cycles) of CPR
Anaphylaxis	Assist person with use of prescribed auto injector
Asthma	Assist person with use of prescribed inhaler

- Check the scene
- Check for responsiveness – ask, "Are you OK?"
- Adult - call 911, then administer CPR
- Child/Infant – administer CPR for 5 cycles, then call 911
- Open victim's airway and check for breathing – look, listen, and feel for 5 - 10 seconds
- Two rescue breaths should be given, 1 second each, and should produce a visible chest rise
- If the air does not go in, reposition and try 2 breaths again
- Check victim's pulse – chest compressions are recommended if an infant or child has a rate less than 60 per minute with signs of poor perfusion.
- Begin 30 compressions to 2 breaths at a rate of 1 breath every 5 seconds for Adult; 1 breath every 3 seconds for child/infant
- Continue 30:2 ratio until victim moves, AED is brought to the scene, or professional help arrives

AED

- ADULT/ Child over 8 years old - use Adult pads
- Child 1-8 years old – use Child pads or use Adult pads by placing one on the chest and one on the back of the child

- Infant under 1 year of age - AED not recommended

Special Report: Guidelines for Standard Precautions

Standard precautions are precautions taken to avoid contracting various diseases and preventing the spread of disease to those who have compromised immunity. Some of these diseases include human immunodeficiency virus (HIV), acquired immunodeficiency syndrome (AIDS), and hepatitis B (HBV). Standard precautions are needed since many diseases do not display signs or symptoms in their early stages. Standard precautions mean to treat all body fluids/ substances as if they were contaminated. These body fluids include but are not limited to the following blood, semen, vaginal secretions, breast milk, amniotic fluid, feces, urine, peritoneal fluid, synovial fluid, cerebrospinal fluid, secretions from the nasal and oral cavities, and lacrimal and sweat gland excretions. This means that standard precautions should be used with all patients.

1. A shield for the eyes and face must be used if there is a possibility of splashes from blood and body fluids.
2. If possibility of blood or body fluids being splashed on clothing, you must wear a plastic apron.
3. Gloves must be worn if you could possibly come in contact with blood or body fluids. They are also needed if you are going to touch something that may have come in contact with blood or body fluids.
4. Hands must be washed even if you were wearing gloves. Hands must be washed and gloves must be changed between patients. Wash hands with at a dime size amount of soap and warm water for about 30 seconds. Singing "Mary had a little lamb" is approximately 30 seconds.
5. Blood and body fluid spills must be cleansed and disinfected using a solution of one part bleach to 10 parts water or your hospital's accepted method.
6. Used needles must be separated from clean needles. Throw both the needle and the syringe away in the sharps' container. The sharps' container is made of puncture proof material.
7. Take extra care in performing high-risk activities that include puncturing the skin and cutting the skin.
8. CPR equipment to be used in a hospital must include resuscitation bags and mouthpieces.

Special precautions must be taken to dispose of biomedical waste. Biomedical waste includes but is not limited to the following: laboratory waste, pathology waste, liquid waste from suction, all sharp object, bladder catheters, chest tubes, IV tubes, and drainage containers. Biomedical waste is removed from a facility by trained biomedical waste disposers.

The health care professional is legally and ethically responsible for adhering to standard precautions. They may prevent you from contracting a fatal disease or from a patient contracting a disease from you that could be deadly.

Special Report: Difficult Patients

Every occupational therapist will eventually get a difficult patient on their list of responsibilities. These patients can be mentally, physically, and emotionally combative in many different environments. Consequently, care of these patients should be conducted in a manner for personal and self-protection of the therapist. Some of the key guidelines are as follows:

1. Never allow yourself to be cornered in a room with the patient positioned between you and the door.
2. Don't escalate the tension with verbal bantering. Basically, don't argue with the patient or resident.
3. Ask permission before performing any normal tasks in a patient's room whenever possible.
4. Discuss your concerns with the nursing staff. Consult the floor supervisor if necessary, especially when safety is an issue.
5. Get help from other support staff when offering care. Get a witness if you are anticipating abuse of any kind.
6. Remove yourself from the situation if you are concerned about your personal safety at all times.
7. If attacked, defend yourself with the force necessary for self-protection and attempt to separate from the patient.
8. Be aware of the patient's medical and mental history prior to entering the patient's room.
9. Don't put yourself in a position to be hurt.
10. Get the necessary help for all transfers, bathing and dressing activities from other staff members for difficult patients.
11. Respect the resident and patient's personal property.
12. Get assistance quickly, via the call bell or vocal projection, if a situation becomes violent or abuse.
13. Immediately seek medical treatment if injured.
14. Fill out an incident report for proper documentation of the occurrence.
15. Protect other patients from abusive behavior.

Special Report: Additional Bonus Material

Due to our efforts to try to keep this book to a manageable length, we've created a link that will give you access to all of your additional bonus material.

Please visit http://www.mometrix.com/bonus948/nbcototr/ to access the information.